# The Law and the Midwife

Rosemary Jenkins

*RGN, RM, MTD, DMS, MBIM*
Formerly Director of Professional Affairs
Royal College of Midwives

**Blackwell
Science**

© 1995 by
Blackwell Science Ltd
Editorial Offices:
Osney Mead, Oxford OX2 0EL
25 John Street, London WC1N 2BL
23 Ainslie Place, Edinburgh EH3 6AJ
238 Main Street, Cambridge,
  Massachusetts 02142, USA
54 University Street, Carlton,
  Victoria 3053, Australia

Other Editorial Offices:
Librairie Arnette SA
1, rue de Lille, 75007 Paris
France

Blackwell Wissenschafts-Verlag GmbH
Kurfürstendamm 57
10707 Berlin, Germany

Blackwell MZV
Feldgasse 13, A-1238 Wien
Austria

First published 1995

Set by DP Photosetting, Aylesbury, Bucks
Printed and bound in Great Britain by
Hartnolls Ltd, Bodmin, Cornwall

DISTRIBUTORS

Marston Book Services Ltd
PO Box 87
Oxford OX2 0DT
(*Orders:* Tel: 01865 791155
         Fax: 01865 791927
         Telex: 837515)

North America
Blackwell Science, Inc.
238 Main Street
Cambridge, MA 02142
(*Orders:* Tel: 800 759-6102
              617 876-7000
         Fax: 617 492-5263)

Australia
Blackwell Science Pty Ltd
54 University Street
Carlton, Victoria 3053
(*Orders:* Tel: (03) 347-5552)

A catalogue record for this book is available
from the British Library

ISBN 0–632–03629–X

Library of Congress
Cataloging in Publication Data
Jenkins, Rosemary.
    The law and the midwife/Rosemary
Jenkins.
       p.   cm.
    Includes bibliographical references and
index.
    ISBN 0-632-03629-X
    1. Midwives—Legal status, laws, etc.—
Great Britain.   I. Title
KD2968.M5J46   1995
344.41′0415—dc20
[341.104415]                    94-23377
                                   CIP

# Contents

# Preface

Why *The Law and the Midwife*? Midwives deliver babies; but it is not as simple as that. They have duties and obligations and others have duties and obligations towards them. Some of those duties are ethical and moral ones, others are required by law. Sometimes the law upholds the moral obligation and sometimes it appears not to be able to provide the answers.

Until just a few years ago the midwife was unlikely to be too aware of the complexities of the various areas of the law as it related to her practice other than the direct requirements of the Midwives Acts and the Rules. Now it is very different. There is an acceptance that medical negligence claims are on the increase and that midwifery and obstetrics are considered 'high risk' for such claims. There have been radical changes in the statutory regulation of the National Health Service (NHS) which have introduced changes to the employment position of the midwife. Very recently greater interest among some midwives in offering their services on a self-employed basis means that the law relating to self-employment and partnership status needs to be considered.

The aim of this book is to take four themes, describe the legal background to them, explain them in the context of midwifery practice and highlight any current debate surrounding them.

These general themes are:

- Midwifery is a profession governed by statute. The history of midwifery legislation, the current position, including a discussion on the interpretation of the Midwives Rules and Code of Practice, and a discussion on the debate over separate midwifery legislation are covered in Chapters 2 and 3.

- The midwife is a professional who, by offering her services, is accountable in law to her client. Chapters 5, 6 and 7 explain the legal duties of the midwife to protect the safety of her clients, to enable them to make appropriate decisions about their care by facilitating their consent to treatment and to ensure confidentiality. Chapter 8 describes some of the statutory rights of pregnant women so that the midwife can help her client in obtaining maximum benefit from these.

- The midwife is commonly an employee and therefore affected by employment law. As she is likely to be an employee of the NHS, which is itself legally constituted, Chapter 4 outlines the history of NHS legislation and describes the present and future situation while Chapter 10 explains briefly employment law.

- The midwife may also be an employer or self-employed in independent practice. Although there are few midwives currently in full independent practice, more who are NHS employees offer limited services outside their employment and there has been a recent upsurge in interest in this form of practice.

To place these themes into a legal context, Chapter 1 outlines some basic legal concepts: what is the law; what legal structures operate; what are the sources of the law; how these in principle apply to midwives. There are fundamental differences between the law in England and Wales and Scottish law, although these are minimal in relation to most of the legal principles discussed in this book. Where differences exist they will be described.

This book has been written by a midwife, not a lawyer. Its intention is not to make lawyers out of midwives but to give them sufficient understanding so that they can make sense of legal principles as these affect their day-to-day work. Part of its intention is to allay many of the anxieties that midwives express about the constraints that they see the law imposing upon them and to enable them to understand that far from constraining, the law frequently operates in such a way as to enable them to extend and develop their practice.

Throughout the book the midwife has been referred to as 'she' and for the sake of clarity, her baby as 'he'.

*Rosemary Jenkins*

# Chapter 1
# The Legal Framework

## WHAT IS THE LAW?

Everyone knows what the law is. It is the 'thing' that enforces speed limits, that prohibits bigamy, that requires punishment for criminal offences and decides what is a criminal offence. It provides a framework for the settlement of disputes. It enables some people to perform certain work activities, for example midwifery, whilst stopping others from doing so. It is not difficult to imagine what the absence of the law would create – lawlessness, anarchy. It is the framework that a society develops to limit lawlessness, thus allowing it to function in a way that is predictable and acceptable to its members. Salmond defines it as 'the body of principles recognised and applied by the State in the administration of justice' [1].

A way of understanding the law is to look first at how the 'body of principles' is developed and then to examine how the legal system administers the law on behalf of the people.

## The derivation of the law

There are three main sources of English law:

- Statute
- Case law
- European law

Scottish Law is also derived from the codified system of Roman Law, but this will not be described in this book as the legal principles affecting midwifery practice are drawn from statute, case law and European law.

## Statutory law

Laws passed by Parliament are the most important source of law. They override decisions made by judges. In terms of the sheer volume, Acts of Parliament also represent the most important source of new law although this has only been the case in this century. Acts of Parliament fulfil certain functions:

1

- They can create new law; for example the Congenital Disabilities (Civil Liability) Act 1976 created a new set of rights for the fetus.

- They can amend existing statutory law; the Nurses, Midwives and Health Visitors Act 1992 made changes to the profession's statutory bodies by amendments to the Nurses, Midwives and Health Visitors Act 1979.

- They can amend, clarify or confirm case law.

- They can repeal existing law.

- They can consolidate a number of disparate laws into one; the Children Act 1989, as well as introducing new legal principles, consolidated all the existing legislation relating to the care of children into the one document, although adoption is still a separate issue.

- They can be enabling; that is the primary legislation allows for secondary legislation or subsequent regulations to fill in the detail of the law without having to be subject to a full debate of Parliament.

An Act of Parliament is confirmed by Royal Assent. However, before this happens there are a number of stages through which it will pass.

When a government is contemplating new legislation it may choose to proceed in various ways. It can, of course, bring the matter immediately to Parliament, but it may choose to seek public opinion first. It may do this with the publication of a Green or a White Paper.

### A Green Paper

A Green Paper is a government consultative document. It is issued when a government wants to elicit a wide range of views before drawing up potential legislation. Not every Bill will be preceded by a Green Paper and not every Green Paper will be followed by legislation. An example of a government Green Paper was the consultation document, published in June 1991, on the Health of the Nation. This proposed ways in which a strategy might be developed to create a healthier population. In fact this document was not converted into legislation but became the Health of the Nation Policy which was launched in mid 1992 [2].

### A White Paper

Whilst a Green Paper is consultative, a White Paper sets out a government's intended policy in a form that enables people to understand it. It uses non-statutory language to describe the contents of an intended Bill. In the past five years three important White Papers were published which led to health care related legislation. *Promoting Better Health*

[3] preceded the Health and Medicines Act 1989; *Working for Patients* [4] and *Caring for People* [5] described the policy that was enacted in the National Health Service and Community Care Act 1990.

Although a White Paper is not a consultation document, it is possible to use the parliamentary process as the subsequent Bill passes through its stages to influence and possibly alter the policy. For example, when the National Health Service and Community Care Bill was being considered by the House of Lords in 1989, the Medical Royal Colleges, the Royal College of Midwives and the Royal College of Nursing lobbied for some caution as they were concerned about the effect the proposed changes would have upon the provision of clinical care. The Government introduced an amendment to the Bill to set up a Clinical Standards Advisory Group, made up of representatives of the Royal Colleges, which would be funded and responsible for monitoring standards of care as the NHS changes were introduced. That Group has reported on such diverse subjects as access to and availability of regional services (including neonatal intensive care) and diabetic services. A report on maternity care is expected in 1994.

### How a Bill becomes an Act

Acts of Parliament are referred to as 'primary legislation'. A proposed Act is firstly presented to the House of Commons (or occasionally to the House of Lords) as a Bill. The Bill then passes through formal stages in both the House of Commons and the House of Lords. These stages are:

(1) **The first reading:** this is a formality, the Bill being introduced to Parliament and its printing ordered.

(2) **The second reading:** this takes the form of a debate on the principles of the proposed legislation. If it passes this stage, the Bill will then pass to the Committee Stage.

(3) **The committee stage.** An all-party committee of the House of Commons, whose membership reflects the composition of the full House, examines the Bill in detail and debates it, clause by clause. At this stage opposition amendments are considered and voted upon. However, as the Committee has the same proportions of Government and Opposition membership as the full House, it is not easy to achieve a successful amendment unless it is either in line with Government policy or a significant number of Government backbenchers are persuaded to oppose their own party.

(4) **The report stage.** The committee reports back to the full House with its recommendations, including any amendments it has considered. At this stage, the Bill passes to the House of Lords.

The Bill passes through the same stages as in the House of Commons although the whole of the House of Lords usually forms the committee for the committee stage.

When all amendments have been agreed by both Houses, the House of Commons takes its final vote and once a majority has voted for the Bill it is given the Royal Assent and becomes an Act, although it may not immediately come into force.

This may seem to be a complicated way for Acts of Parliament to be enacted but much legislation is not controversial and these stages can be passed over very quickly. All primary legislation, however, needs parliamentary time and it would be impossible for Parliament to consider every detail of proposed law. Much law is very technical; setting revised speed limits or motorway regulations, for example. To deal with the mass of technical law, much primary legislation is now 'enabling' and delegates authority to a Minister to introduce detailed secondary legislation.

### Secondary legislation

Secondary or delegated legislation is derived from powers set out in primary legislation and takes the form of statutory instruments. The advantage of using secondary legislation is that, with the highly technical nature of some laws today, they can be drawn up and approved by experts and, if they require subsequent amendment, this does not have to wait, sometimes for a considerable period, for parliamentary time.

A good example of how this system works is the Midwives Rules. These Rules are a statutory instrument and the primary legislation is the Nurses, Midwives and Health Visitors Act 1979. This Act gives to the United Kingdom Central Council for Nurses, Midwives and Health Visitors (UKCC) the power to draw up the Midwives Rules and amend them as necessary. The UKCC does this from time to time in consultation with its Midwifery Committee, thus using the expertise of practising midwives to frame the legislation. Once agreed, the Secretary of State, in this case for Health, endorses the legislation by laying it before the House of Commons for automatic approval.

## Other parliamentary processes

Before moving on to discuss other sources of law, there are some other parliamentary processes that are important even though they do not in themselves produce legislation.

### Parliamentary select committees

This is a system of committees of parliamentary back-benchers which 'mirror' the major government departments. There are, for example, committees for Defence, Social Security and Agriculture. There is a Health Select Committee. Each committee has a chairman, elected by its members, and comprises members from various parties although the overall membership reflects the current composition of Parliament. Thus the party in power will always constitute the majority on any committee.

These committees have no statutory function although they can exercise an influence over policy. They also have the power to question Ministers about past Government action, about present policy and about future Government intentions. Their hearings are public and the evidence they obtain both in writing and verbally is published.

They have complete freedom over the topics they want to study, although they are often influenced by current matters of controversy, and when conducting any enquiry they invite evidence from a wide range of sources. They are also able to make visits if they believe this will aid their final recommendations. When they are considering matters of a technical nature, they almost always appoint a panel of advisers to assist them in their enquiry. There have been a number of influential reports on maternity services from the committee concerned (originally called the Social Services Committee and now the Health Committee). In 1980 the Short Report (the chairman was then Renée Short MP) followed an enquiry into perinatal mortality [6]. The Winterton Report (chairman, Nicholas Winterton MP) resulted from a year spent looking at the general provision of maternity services [7].

Select Committee hearings are open to the public. The times and subjects to be discussed are listed in most of the national 'broadsheet' newspapers at the beginning of the week. The room number where the hearing is to take place is also given and entry to the House of Commons is via the main public entrance. Midwives wishing to attend one of these hearings should avoid the public queue and present themselves to the policemen at the entrance. They will get immediate entry.

### Specific parliamentary enquiries

Not all parliamentary reports emanate from the select committee process. Ministers may order an enquiry if they believe there is a matter of public interest. As an example, following publication of the Winterton Report in 1992 the Government set up an expert working group chaired by the Junior Health Minister, Baroness Cumberlege, to examine the implications of the radical recommendations that the report had outlined. The result of that enquiry was published in 1993, the policy document *Changing Childbirth* [8].

### Parliamentary questions and early day motions.

Government ministers are accountable to Parliament and to their back-benchers for what they do. There are two mechanisms that MPs can use to call ministers to account. Ministers must answer questions put to them by MPs when asked as a 'parliamentary question'. The answers can be given verbally in Parliament or as a written answer.

Alternatively, motions can be laid before Parliament. These are placed at the Dispatch Box and individual MPs can then sign them if they support the principle. If sufficient MPs sign an 'early day motion', as it is called, indicating general support of the House, the Government may consider legislation to support the principle.

The following is a parliamentary question which was asked in 1991 during the Health Committee enquiry.

'To ask the Secretary of State for Health what is her policy on home confinements.'

To which the reply was given

'Although the demand for home births is not great, health authorities should ensure that there are policies agreed between the professionals to provide mothers who do decide to have their babies at home with adequate antenatal, intrapartum and postnatal care and that these arrangements are well known locally.'

Parliamentary questions and early day motions on their own are not very influential in shaping government policy and legislation. However, they can be used in conjunction with parliamentary lobbying and other forms of public pressure to influence statutory law.

Another small but important use of the parliamentary question is to obtain information that would usually take time to research. An example of this was the question asked in April 1994:

'To ask the Secretary of State for Health if she will list those Trusts, by region, that have failed to achieve a capital return of 6% or more . . .'

### The Private Members' Bill

Ordinary MPs may bring their own Bills before Parliament. This is a difficult procedure as they are allotted parliamentary time on the basis of a ballot. There are occasions when issues of important ethical implication are eventually made law through this process. There are some issues that political parties prefer not to support but which nevertheless require statutory support and the Private Members' Bill may be the only way to achieve this. The notable example of this was the Abortion Act 1967, introduced by David Steel. Although the 'lottery' of a parliamentary ballot means that this type of legislation is not easily achieved, MPs sometimes win parliamentary time first and subsequently choose a subject to put forward. This can be an ideal opportunity to lobby the fortunate MP to take up a particular cause.

## Case law

Until the twentieth century the most important source of English law was case law or common law. This is the legal framework that is based upon the decisions of judges. There are certain rules that apply to the development and subsequent use of case law which can be summarized under the general description of precedent.

First, a judge usually follows the decision of a previous court hearing. This rule results in a degree of certainty about the eventual outcome of future cases. It is, however, possible for a judge to determine that the case he is currently hearing differs in some respect from previous decisions, or 'distinguish' it, allowing him to make a fresh judgment. If he does this he should, in summing up the case, state why he has come to the decision he has. Significantly the House of Lords may depart from a previous decision when it appears right to do so but this is not a step that is taken lightly.

Secondly, a judge in a lower court is absolutely bound to follow decisions made in a higher court. A judge in a County Court, therefore may not go against a decision made in a similar case in the High Court or the Court of Appeal go against the House of Lords.

Case law can fulfil three main objectives:

(1) It can be used to introduce a completely new legal principle. The law on negligence (which will be covered in Chapter 5) was finally defined by a decision of the House of Lords on the Scottish case, *Donoghue* v. *Stevenson* (1932).

(2) It can be used to develop existing law. An example of this is the *Bolam* test (described further in Chapter 5) where a judgment was made which determined the professional standard that should be met when deciding whether a professional person had been negligent or not. In this case, the law of negligence already existed and the judgment merely clarified it.

(3) It can be used to clarify the terms of a statute. Although the wording of all Acts of Parliament is carefully drafted, there can still be ambiguities. An example of this is Section 17(1) of the Nurses, Midwives and Health Visitors Act 1979. It states 'A person other than a registered midwife or a registered medical practitioner shall

not attend a women in childbirth'. There is no clarity about either the words 'attend' or 'childbirth'. Does 'attend' mean to be there or to offer professional services; is 'childbirth' just the delivery, is it labour as well or does it extend to the whole process and include pregnancy? It may not be necessary or desirable to define with clarity what these mean, but the only way a precise definition could become law would be if a judge hearing a relevant case offered a judicial definition.

Legal cases are reported through a number of official law reports and when lawyers are trying to decide what the outcome of a case might be they refer to these. They will be looking for what the judges have said. Judgments consist of two parts. The first is the actual judgment, and if made in a superior court this will act as precedent and further decisions will have to follow it. The judge, in any case, may also make subsidiary remarks, particularly explaining why he made the decisions he did. These statements may also influence future judgments but are not mandatory. It is also the case that some past judgments may seem to be contradictory or poorly 'distinguished'. For these reasons, the rules of precedent, which evolved to ensure a degree of certainty about the outcome of a case, still leave some doubt about the decision a judge will make in any case before him.

# European law

Although statutory law holds precedence over all other sources of law derived in the UK, since entry into the European Union, Community law can now override law made by judges and Parliament.

### Regulations and Directives

The Council of Ministers and the European Commission make laws known as Regulations and Directives. It should be noted that the elected European Parliament plays a minor role in the determination of European law although it was somewhat strengthened by the Maastricht Treaty of 1991.

A Regulation is 'binding in its entirety and directly applicable in all member states' and a Directive is 'binding as to the result to be achieved' but member states may decide for themselves on the best way of achieving the Directive's requirements. Once a Directive is agreed the participating countries are expected to incorporate the terms of the agreement into their own legislation. This mechanism is demonstrated by the acceptance of the Midwives Directive into the UK Midwives Rules and into the requirements for midwifery training. Rule 33(3)(a) states that UK programmes of midwifery education must 'meet the requirements of the Midwives Directive'.

If some part of intended European legislation is unacceptable to one of the countries, it is usual for that country to seek exemption within the terms of the Directive rather than subsequently ignore the Directive once passed. The British government therefore sought exemption from what it saw as some of the more restricting clauses of the Social Chapter.

## The European Court of Justice

The European Court of Justice, based in Luxembourg, has responsibility for deciding disputes arising from the various treaties that exist between the members of the European Union. It is the supreme court in these matters. Lord Denning stated in a 1974 judgment (*H.P. Bulmer Ltd* v. *J. Bollinger SA*):

> 'In the task of interpreting the Treaty, the English judges are no longer the final authority . . . The supreme tribunal for interpreting the Treaty is the European Court of Justice at Luxembourg.'

The Court consists of one judge from each member state. Their decisions apply both to the arbitration between parties in dispute (governments, institutions, companies or individuals) and to the authoritative interpretation of the European law.

## The European Court of Human Rights

This court, which is based in Strasbourg, was set up after the 1950 Convention on Human Rights to which the UK was a signatory. It is possible for people who are dissatisfied with decisions made by UK courts to petition the European Commission on Human Rights. Any unresolved disputes will be heard by the Court of Human Rights.

## The EC Advisory Committee on the Training of Midwives

This is a permanent committee which has a responsibility to monitor the working of the Midwives Directive. Each member state has three midwife representatives on the committee, one for clinical practice, one for education and one for the 'competent body' (in the UK the UKCC). Each of these representatives has a named alternate to attend meetings when she is not able to. The membership in the UK is allocated so that all the component countries are represented.

# Natural justice

The principles of natural justice are not in themselves sources of law.

However certain rights of justice are accepted as rules to guide any adjudication on matters in dispute. The main concepts of natural justice are:

- to act fairly and in good faith;
- to allow each party the opportunity to state his case adequately;
- that a man must not be judge in his own case;
- that a person must be told of what he is accused; and
- that all documents used in the adjudication process must be available to both the parties.

In summary, these rules could be stated as 'justice should not only be done but be seen to be done'.

Where it is alleged that the actions of a public body may be in contravention of natural justice, it can be possible to apply to the High Court for a judicial review. For example the midwife, Jilly Rosser, used the judicial review process when she claimed that her case had been unfairly heard by the Professional Conduct Committee of the UKCC. The High Court case here was not concluded because the UKCC accepted irregularities in the original hearing and overturned the decision of the Professional Conduct Committee so that a final judgment was not necessary.

## THE STRUCTURE OF THE LAW

Very generally the law can be divided into two divisions; public law (which includes criminal, constitutional and administrative law) and private, or civil law (which includes the law on negligence, contract and family law). A 'rule of thumb' definition is that the civil law deals with disputes that occur between individuals whereas the public law deals with disputes between an individual and society or the organs of society. There are occasions when it is not always easy to determine the difference between them. For example assault can be a criminal offence or a civil wrong. It is often easier to define some of the different ways which the two systems operate rather than define the two systems.

- There are separate court systems depending upon whether the case is a civil or a criminal case.

- There is a different burden of proof in the two systems. In the criminal system proof has to be 'beyond a reasonable doubt' whereas in the civil system judgments are made 'on the balance of probabilities'.

- The sanctions are also different. The criminal system seeks to punish and to remove those who are a danger to society by, for example, giving custodial sentences. The civil system seeks to redress a wrong by awarding damages, or seeks to stop a wrong being perpetrated through the issuing of injunctions.

- The processes of civil and criminal actions also differ as they pass through the parallel court systems.

# Civil law

Civil law encompasses a number of different areas of the law; contract law, some of which relates to employment law; specialized commercial law; family law; the law of property.

## The process of a civil action

Most of the actions taken out against health authorities or professionals are civil cases, seeking to redress an alleged civil wrong. The rules of procedure involve considerable legal activity prior to a court hearing. This is conducted by the lawyers representing the parties to the case. The person who brings an action is called the plaintiff and the person or body answering the allegation, the defendant.

The pre-court proceedings start with a notification that a potential claim may be brought and asking for any papers that may relate to the case. All relevant papers must be forwarded to the plaintiff's legal representatives. An official notification of an intended case (a writ) is sent to the court which then requires the lawyers to enter the relevant papers. At this stage it is usual for the lawyers to meet in order to attempt to achieve a settlement of the dispute without the necessity for a court hearing. Most cases are concluded during this out-of-court negotiating period. This pre-hearing activity is also important to ensure that the elements of the dispute between the parties are very clearly defined and all supporting evidence has been identified before going to court. This saves court time.

## The structure of the civil courts

The court system is hierarchical with lesser cases going to the lower courts and the opportunity to appeal then being through the higher courts. Claims of a small nature are heard at the County Court level but most obstetric claims are of a serious nature and will be referred to the High Court in the Queen's Bench Division. Appeals from both the County Court and the High Court are referred to the Court of Appeal (Civil Division) although some cases are able to 'leap-frog' to appeal directly to the House of Lords.

Since the UK entered the European Community in 1973 it has been possible to have leave to appeal to the European Court of Justice. Not

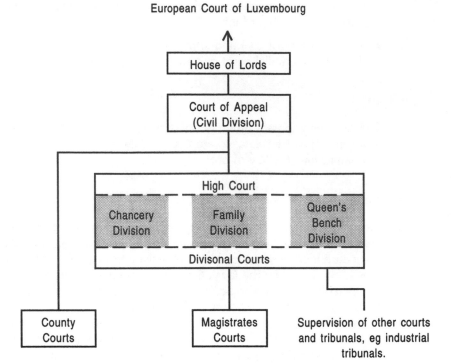

**Fig. 1.1** The civil court system.

all cases are allowed to go to this level, but if there is an important issue of European law to be decided the case is usually referred.

## Public law

### The criminal court system

Like the civil courts, the criminal courts operate as a hierarchy, with lesser cases being heard by the Magistrates' Courts and more serious cases going to the Crown Court. There is a similar appeal mechanism to the Court of Appeal (Criminal Division) and through to the House of Lords. Leave must be granted for a case to go forward for appeal and the appeal takes the form of a review of the reports of the case, the case not being heard again. It is also possible for the prosecution to appeal against sentencing if it believes it is too lenient. It is fortunately rare for cases relating to the provision of health care to be the subject of criminal proceedings.

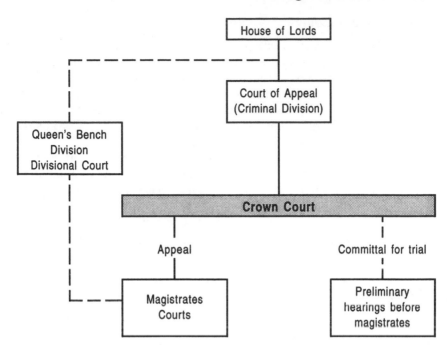

**Fig. 1.2** The criminal court systems.

## Constitutional law

This part of the public law covers cases where the mechanisms of the state are involved, including the law relating to welfare services, public corporations and the functions of local government.

It is of fundamental importance in that it incorporates the rights and liberties of the individual within the state. These civil liberties include:

- the right to personal freedom (a person may not be imprisoned without justification);
- the right to freedom of speech (the right to write or say anything as long as it does not infringe the law);
- the right to freedom of movement;
- the right to practise religion; and
- the right to vote.

In general, where an individual believes he has been deprived of his civil liberties or where an administrative decision appears to have been made in breach of the principles of natural justice it may be possible to apply to the High Court to seek redress through the process of judicial review.

### The Coroner's Court

The Coroner is an officer of the Crown who has a duty to inquire into the cause of death of anyone who is killed or dies in suspicious circumstances. Suspicious circumstances are defined fairly broadly so that some deaths in hospital may be referred to a Coroner's Court. The Coroner usually sits alone but in some circumstances may or must have a jury with him to support the decision of the court. A Coroner must be either medically or legally qualified.

People who are required to attend a Coroner's Court do so as witnesses. As such they are not entitled to representation although any midwife finding herself in this situation may want to take someone from her professional organization with her to give support.

The Coroner confines his judgment to the cause of death and does not apportion blame to any person. However, his judgment may lead directly to criminal charges and a subsequent trial.

## Tribunals

As well as the criminal and civil courts there are various tribunals that operate in the legal system. They are often technical in their nature – Industrial Tribunals, Medical Appeals Tribunals, Supplementary Benefit Appeals Tribunals, Rent Tribunals – and as such draw upon experts in their field to sit on the adjudicating panel. The chairman may or may not be a lawyer. The function of a tribunal is to adjudicate in a dispute without using the full complexity of the law. They are usually much cheaper to operate and a resolution to a dispute is reached more quickly. Appeal against a tribunal decision can usually only be made on a point of law rather than on the facts of the case.

## Legal personnel

**Solicitors.** Solicitors offer a full range of legal services and advice. Many of them specialize in chosen areas of the law including some in health service related work. As well as giving direct advice, solicitors usually prepare the preliminary brief for cases which will be heard in court. Until recently they were barred from right of audience (that is, to argue a case) in all but the lowest courts but this has now been relaxed. It is also now possible, although not yet common, for a solicitor to be appointed as a lower court judge.

**Barristers.** After legal training and pupillage, a barrister becomes a member of one of the four Inns of Court. They have right of audience in all levels of the court systems. After some time in practice they may be appointed Queen's Counsel. Most of the judges, and all of the senior judges, are appointed from the practising barristers.

**The Lord Chancellor.** This is the highest legal office in the British constitution. He is a Privy Councillor, President of the House of Lords and a member of the Cabinet. He appoints magistrates and circuit judges and nominates the High Court judges.

## Legal aid

Legal aid is the system of financial assistance given to help people to take a dispute to court. Its usefulness is however extremely limited as it is means tested and only those on very low incomes can qualify. As most legal actions are potentially very costly, only those who are rich enough to be able to afford to pay, or those poor enough for legal aid can use the court system. There are however two exceptions to this.

For the purposes of legal aid, a child is assessed on his own finances if through a 'friend' he wishes to go to court. As very few children have an income of their own, this effectively means that use of legal aid is open to children. Particularly, in relation to the maternity services, a baby has almost unlimited access to the legal system so that financial constraints need not be considered if a negligence claim is being contemplated.

The second way in which people can occasionally gain access to the legal system is to find a 'backer' who will assist them with it. Organizations may wish to clarify or change the existing law by helping someone to take a 'test-case'. Particularly active in this is the Equal Opportunities Commission which has supported cases, even to the European Court of Justice, in order to clarify the equal opportunities legislation.

## The legal system in Scotland

The principal law officer of the Crown in Scotland is the Lord Advocate. It is customary for him to hold a seat in one of the Houses of Parliament and he is a UK Minister with special responsibilities for Scotland. It is a government appointment so that he leaves office if the government changes. He is responsible for the investigation of crime in Scotland and for prosecutions in the High Court. He is also responsible for drafting Scottish legislation and acts as constitutional and legal adviser to the government.

The Procurators Fiscal are the law officers responsible for prosecutions in every Sheriff and District Court. They also investigate all suspicious deaths as there is no office of Coroner in Scotland.

The court system in Scotland also differs from the English system. The highest criminal court is the High Court of Justiciary which also sits, with three judges, as the Court of Criminal Appeal. There is no right of criminal appeal to the House of Lords. Under this level, Scotland is divided into six sheriffdoms, each with a Sheriff Court and a Sheriff Principal. These in turn are divided into 49 districts with District Courts. These equate with the Magistrates' Courts in England and Wales and the bench is made up of Justices of the Peace.

The highest civil court in Scotland is the Court of Session from which there is a right of appeal to the House of Lords. The Sheriff Courts deal with most of the civil litigation in Scotland.

## USING THE LEGAL PROCESSES

### The system of government

The British system of government is a parliamentary democracy. The people are represented through their elected MPs and this is done on a constituency basis. Most of these members will be ordinary MPs although a few will be Ministers of State and fewer still will be Secretaries of State and members of the Cabinet. Ministers and Secretaries of State, with the Prime Minister, form the Government, whilst the ordinary MPs form Parliament. The Government is responsible to Parliament for the development of policy and legislation.

Also supporting Government, and influential in policy formulation and implementation is the Civil Service. Roughly, this is divided into departments or offices that support each Secretary of State.

### Lobbying for change

Although it is theoretically possible for UK citizens to influence the law-making process through contact with local MPs, this is in reality a very difficult process. Members of Parliament usually hold local 'surgeries' that are advertised in the press. Their time is limited, however, and they have to listen to many competing interests. They also have interests of their own and of their party, as well as a need to satisfy majority wishes so that they are in a strong position at election time. It usually needs a concerted and nationally led effort to bring pressure to bear on a busy Government and Parliament. This can be done by setting up special interest pressure groups. Many of the established charities act in this capacity. Charities such as MIND and Age Concern represent the interests of some of the most vulnerable members of society by meeting with Ministers and MPs and by working with and advising Parliamentary Select Committees and the Civil Service.

To explain how a successful campaign can be run, the following case study demonstrates the time, patience and commitment needed.

## Case study: changing maternity policy

### The background

For some decades during and after the Second World War there had been a slow change in maternity care with more women choosing to have their babies in hospital. The system still accommodated the wishes of women to have their babies at home, whilst those midwives who worked in hospital still practised in an autonomous manner, working as colleagues with the obstetrician. Up to the late 1960s there was still a network of smaller maternity homes and units where a woman could chose to have her baby. In 1970 a Government supported committee under the chairmanship of Sir John Peel reported on the maternity services. The report, *Domiciliary Midwifery and Maternity Bed Needs* [9], recommended that sufficient facilities should be made available for all women to deliver in consultant led units. This coincided with a variety of technical developments, electronic fetal monitoring and ultrasound scanning, and, encouraged by Government policy and generous funding, almost 100% delivery in hospital was achieved in the space of a few years. Doctors took control of the technological developments and the midwife rapidly lost her autonomy. Midwifery was not organized at the time and many felt that it would disappear as a separate profession.

As an indicator of the weak position of the midwife, it was the women, through organizations such as the National Childbirth Trust (NCT) and the Association for Improvements in Maternity Services (AIMS) who began to challenge the situation.

At the beginning of the 1980s the Select Committee for Health and Social Services produced a number of influential reports. They were advised by obstetricians and, not surprisingly, their reports supported the investment in technology even though they acknowledged that maternity care needed to become more 'human' and cater for women's social and emotional needs. Universal hospital delivery was supported. More and more women found it difficult to have a homebirth and many of the smaller maternity units were closed down as large, hospital based, consultant led units were opened.

### The present situation

Although the current provision of maternity services has not altered from the reliance upon consultant led hospital care, there has been a major change in Government and Parliamentary policy. In 1992 the Health Select Committee reported its recommendations after a year long study of maternity care. It concluded that choice for women should be available and that the midwife was the best-placed professional to be able to facilitate this. A subsequent Government working party has endorsed this finding and the NHS has been instructed to re-focus maternity care. The 'political' emergence of midwifery has probably played a great part in this policy U-turn.

### How it was done

First, a pressure group had been formed, the Association of Radical Midwives. It was and continues to be a relatively small and underfunded group, but it began to debate, publicly, some of the problems faced by midwives and to offer some solutions.

One of the continuing strengths of the profession was the loyalty towards the Royal College of Midwives. The organization has always enjoyed a high level of membership and thus has been able to claim it represents the majority view. In the mid 1980s the College began to use this power to influence Government.

It began to adopt some very simple messages:

● that women should have greater choice in childbirth;
● that the midwife should be able to practise autonomously in giving care to women with uncomplicated pregnancies;
● that the duplication of care that existed between midwife, general practitioner and obstetrician should be stopped; and
● that the focus of care should shift to the community.

To assist in promoting these messages, the College appointed a parliamentary and press officer and began an information campaign. It encouraged its branches to hold meetings before the general election in 1987. It targeted all new MPs after the election with its 'manifesto' for maternity care. It approached a few MPs who agreed to act as an informal panel, raising matters concerning midwives in Parliament. It began to make regular contact with the national press through press releases and press conferences. It also began to train a network of local branch press officers who began to raise the profile of the midwife through the local press. In short it began to enhance the image of the midwife and of the College itself.

### The results

The campaign produced slow but powerful results. When the Select Committee decided to look at maternity services again it invited two midwives to advise it alongside doctors. A midwife had an equal place on the subsequent Government working party which produced the consultative document, *Changing Childbirth*. There is no doubt midwives will now be fully involved in making the changes happen.

In summary, the lesson to be drawn from this case study is that changes in Government policy can be achieved, using the parliamentary system if:

● there is a very clear purpose or message which is supported throughout any campaign;
● the media is fully exploited to disseminate the message of the campaign;
● there is clearly focussed activity at national and local level; and
● campaign 'experts' are used.

## Influencing consultation processes

Earlier in this chapter Green and White Papers were described. The Green Paper is a consultation document, a White Paper enables influence to be directed to MPs as a Bill passes through Parliament. Consultation papers are also sent from the Department of Health and from the National Health Service Executive. In many cases the result of these consultations will be incorporated into either formal legislation or into policy.

A current example of this is the consultation document, *Managing the New National Health Service* [10]. The Government intends to remove the statutory nature of Regional Health Authorities in 1996 and is consulting at the moment about how the process should take place and on what are seen as the main implications of such a change. This is an important consultation for midwives to be involved in as Regional Health Authorities at present have responsibility for the overall provision of midwifery training and have a statutory responsibility for the supervision of midwives. The opportunity should be taken to influence any future change early in the proceedings. At the moment it is unclear when the Bill will be presented to Parliament due to limitations upon parliamentary time for debate.

## SUMMARY

This chapter has outlined the processes and structure of the law in the UK. This will form the basis for understanding how some of the specific areas of law that are covered in later chapters have come about.

Understanding a little of the parliamentary process will enable midwives to take the opportunities, when available, to influence Government policy and legislation.

## FURTHER ACTION

- Attend a session of Parliament or a select committee hearing.

- Find out when your local MP holds a 'surgery'.

## REFERENCES

1. Salmond in Rutherford L., Bone, S. (eds). *Osborn's Concise Law Dictionary*, 8th edn, London. Sweet and Maxwell, 1993.
2. Department of Health. *The Health of the Nation: a strategy for health in England*. London, HMSO, 1992.
3. Department of Health and Social Services. *Promoting Better Health: the Government's programme for improving primary health care*. London, HMSO, 1987.

4. Department of Health. *Working for Patients*. London, HMSO, 1989.
5. Department of Health. *Caring for People: community care in the next decade and beyond*. London, HMSO, 1990.
6. Parliamentary Report of the House of Commons Social Services Committee. *Perinatal and Neonatal Mortality*. Second Report, Session 1979–80, Vol. 1. London, HMSO, 1980.
7. Parliamentary Report of the House of Commons Health Committee. *Maternity Services*. Second Report, Session 1991–92, Vol. 1. London, HMSO, 1992.
8. Department of Health. *Changing Childbirth*. London, HMSO, 1993.
9. Department of Health and Social Security. *Domiciliary Midwifery and Maternity Bed Needs*. London, HMSO, 1970.
10. National Health Service Management Executive. *Managing the New NHS*. Leeds NHSME, 1993.

# Chapter 2
# The Statutory Profession of Midwifery

Almost all the occupations considered professions are in some way controlled by statute. The Medical Act was first passed in 1858; solicitors are governed by the Solicitors Act 1974.

## HISTORY OF MIDWIFERY LEGISLATION

The previous chapter outlined the effort needed to influence legislation. It takes considerable, planned activity and change is rarely achieved rapidly. This was certainly the case for the group of women who took just over 20 years to campaign for a Midwives Act. The history of this fascinating period is better described elsewhere [1]. It is worth noting that they followed the same principles as outlined in Chapter 1. They had a single goal, they organized themselves (as the Midwives Institute, which later became the Royal College of Midwives) and they targeted the people with influence. They had opposition from the medical profession and from the nurses but by arguing that a well trained profession could improve the health of mothers and their babies they were successful.

### The Midwives Act 1902

This first Midwives Act received Royal Assent on 31 July 1902. Figure 2.1 shows the front page of this Act. The first of its clauses stated:

'From and after the first day of April one thousand nine hundred and five, any woman who not being certified under this Act shall take or use the name or title of midwife (either alone or in combination with any other word or words), or any name, title, addition, or description implying that she is certified under this Act, or is a person specially qualified to practise midwifery, or is recognised by law as a midwife, shall be liable on summary conviction to a fine not exceeding five pounds.'

This first Act applied only to England and Wales and its main provi-

21

# Midwives Act, 1902
## [2 EDW. 7. CH. 17.]

### ARRANGEMENT OF SECTIONS.

A.D.
1902.

*[Price 3d. Net.]*     A          i

Fig. 2.1 The front page of the Midwives Act 1902.

sion was to set up a statutory body for midwives, the Central Midwives Board.

The original membership of the Board reflected the difficulties experienced and the compromises that were eventually made in order to achieve the legislation. Midwives were very much in the minority. The membership was made up of:

- four registered medical practitioners, one to be appointed by the Royal College of Physicians of London, one by the Royal College of Surgeons of England, one by the Society of Apothecaries and one by the Incorporated Midwives Institute; and

- two persons (one of whom was to be a woman) to be appointed for terms of three years by the Lord President of the Council; and

- one person to be appointed for a term of three years by the Association of County Councils; and

- one person to be appointed for a term of three years by the Queen Victoria's Jubilee Institute for Nurses; and

- one person to be appointed for a term of three years by the Royal British Nurses Association.

The first Board members were:

| | |
|---|---|
| Dr Champneys | Royal College of Physicians |
| Mr Ward Cousins | Royal College of Surgeons |
| Dr Parker Young | Society of Apothecaries |
| Dr Cullingworth | Incorporated Midwives Institute |
| Dr Sinclair | Privy Council |
| Miss Jane Wilson | |
| Mr Heywood Johnstone | Association of County Councils |
| Miss Rosalind Paget | Queen Victoria's Jubilee Institute for Nurses |
| Miss Oldham | Royal British Nurses' Association |

Powers given to the Central Midwives Board by the legislation were:

(1) to frame rules:
   (a) regulating their own proceedings,
   (b) regulating the issue of certificates and the condition of admission to the Roll of Midwives,
   (c) regulating the course of training, the conduct of examinations and the remuneration of examiners,

(d) regulating the admission to the Roll of women already in practice as midwives at the passing of the Act,

(e) regulating, supervising and restricting within due limits the practice of midwives,

(f) deciding the conditions under which midwives might be suspended from practice,

(g) defining the particulars required to be given in any notice under section 10 of the Act (which required the notification of intention to practise);

(2) to appoint examiners;

(3) to decide upon the place where and the time when examinations should be held;

(4) to publish annually a Roll of Midwives who had been duly certified under the Act;

(5) to decide upon the removal from the Roll of the name of any midwife for disobeying the rules and regulations from time to time laid down under the Act by the Central Midwives Board, or for other misconduct, and also to decide upon the restoration to the Roll of the name of any midwife so removed;

(6) to issue and cancel certificates; and

(7) generally to do any other act or duty which might be necessary for the due and proper carrying out of the provisions of the Act.

One of the first tasks of the Board was to establish the Roll of Midwives. The criteria for entry to the Roll were that the midwife should:

(1) be in possession of a recognised qualification in midwifery, the certificate of the London Obstetrical Society being one of the acceptable qualifications; or

(2) have been in *bona fide* (genuine) practice as a midwife for one year and be of good character; or

(3) meet the requirements of the Board for training and examinations.

## The Midwives Rules – early versions

The Board then set about formulating rules for the practice and training of midwives. The first set of Midwives Rules was issued in 1903. They laid emphasis on cleanliness in practice. One of the rules in the 1919 version could almost be used for today's advice on protection against blood borne diseases.

'The midwife must be scrupulously clean in every way, including her person, clothing, appliances and house; she must keep her nails cut short, and preserve the skin of her hands as far as possible from cracks and abrasions.'

The 1919 version also set out the requirements for summoning medical aid which the midwife was required to do 'in all cases of illness of the patient or child, or of any abnormality occurring during pregnancy, labour or lying-in'. A list of the conditions was then given for which this rule would apply (Figure 2.2).

It is interesting to compare them with our current knowledge about what constitutes an abnormality. With one or two exceptions, the problems are the same it is only the magnitude of them that is different. The main difference is the absence of fetal problems.

Another gem in this version of the Rules is found in the section requiring midwives to make various notifications to the local supervising authority (LSA). Along with notifications when medical aid had been sought, and on the death of a mother or child and all stillbirths, there was one that required the midwife to notify the LSA 'whenever it is proposed to substitute artificial feeding for breast feeding.'

In 1902 midwives worked as independent practitioners so the Board considered ways in which it could enforce compliance with its Rules. It set up a system of supervision of the practising midwife. The origins and subsequent development of this unique form of professional regulation are covered in the next chapter.

## Subsequent enactments

The Central Midwives Board set up by the 1902 Act covered England and Wales only. In 1915 the Midwives (Scotland) Act was passed followed by the Midwives Act (Ireland) in 1918. When Ireland was partitioned in 1922 a Joint Nurses and Midwives Council (Northern Ireland) Act set up a joint statutory body for the two professions.

There have been a number of Midwives Acts since 1902 but most have introduced minor amendments or have been consolidating legislation. The only major change to have been introduced between 1902 and 1979 was the 1936 Act which introduced a salaried midwifery service – local authorities would be responsible for the provision of a midwifery service and midwives would be their employees.

Section 1 of that Act (which incidentally amended the previous Midwives Acts rather than creating a whole new Act) stated,

'It shall be the duty of every local supervising authority within the meaning of the principal Act ... to secure, whether by making arrangements with welfare councils or voluntary organisations for the

26

*21.The foregoing rule shall particularly apply :—

(1) In all cases in which a woman during PREGNANCY, LABOUR, or LYING-IN appears to be dying or is dead.

PREGNANCY.

(2) In the case of a Pregnant woman, when there is any abnormality or complication, such as—

Deformity or stunted growth,

Loss of blood,

Abortion or threatened Abortion,

Excessive sickness,

Puffiness of hands or face,

Fits or Convulsions,

Dangerous varicose veins,

Purulent discharge,

Sores of the genitals.

LABOUR.

(3) In the case of a woman in Labour at or near term, when there is any abnormality of complication, such as—

Fits or Convulsions,

A purulent discharge,

Sores of the genitals,

A malpresentation,

Presentation other than the uncomplicated head or breech,

Where no presentation can be made out,

Where there is excessive bleeding,

\* See Rule 26.

**Fig. 2.2** An extract from the 1919 Midwives Rules.

27

Where two hours after the birth of the child the placenta and membranes have not been completely expelled,

In cases of serious rupture of the perinaeum, or of other injuries of the soft parts.

## LYING-IN.

(4) In the case of a LYING-IN woman, when there is any abnormality or complication, such as—

Fits or Convulsions,

Abdominal swelling and tenderness,

Offensive lochia, if persistent,

Rigor, with raised temperature,

Rise of temperature above **100.4°F.** with quickening of the pulse, for more than twenty-four hours,

Unusual swelling of the breasts with local tenderness or pain,

Secondary post-partum hæmorrhage,

White leg.

## THE CHILD.

(5) In the case of the Child, when there is any abnormality or complication, such as—

Injuries received during birth,

Any malformation or deformity endangering the child's life,

Dangerous feebleness,

†Inflammation of, or discharge from, the eyes, however slight,

† *Note.*—In cases where the eyes are affected the duties of the midwife are :—

(1) Immediately to advise medical help.

(2) To fill up and hand to the nearest relative or friend the form for medical help (see Rules *E* 20 and 23 (*a*).

(3) To send notice to the Local Supervising Authority that medical help has been sought (see Rules *E* 22 (I) (*a*) and 23 (*a*)).

(4) **Also** when there is a **purulent** discharge commencing within 21 days from the date of birth and medical help has **not** been obtained for this discharge, to notify the Local Sanitary Authority. (See Rule *E* 6, *Note.*)

employment by those councils or organisations of certified midwives as whole time servants or by itself employing such midwives, that the number of certified midwives so employed who are available in its area for attendance on women in their own homes as midwives or as maternity nurses during childbirth and from time to time thereafter during a period not less than the lying-in period, is adequate for the needs of the area.'

This was of course prior to the NHS so there was no such statutory provision for hospital care. Midwives were however employed in the voluntary and private hospital sectors. After 1936 some midwives still continued to offer their services for a fee, but many sought the relative stability of paid employment and working in the independent sector became increasingly precarious.

The Midwives Act 1951 consolidated all the previous Midwives Acts and amendments into one. It did not, however, introduce any major change in the statutory position of the midwife, and the statutory framework remained in place until the passage of the Nurses, Midwives and Health Visitors Act 1979.

## Report of the Committee on Nursing (the Briggs Report)

In 1970 a committee was set up under the chairmanship of Professor Asa Briggs. It had as its terms of reference

'To review the role of the nurse and the midwife in the hospital and the community and the education and training required for that role, so that the best use is made of available manpower to meet present needs and the needs of an integrated health service'.

The report [2] was presented to Parliament by the Secretaries of State for Social Services, for Scotland and for Wales. It therefore applied also to these countries.

The report made many far-reaching recommendations, some of which have been taken up subsequently. Many were, as the terms of reference indicate, about the provision of education but some referred to the statutory framework for the professions.

The Committee said,

'At present there is a wide range of bodies concerned with nursing and midwifery education and directly or indirectly, therefore, with the future of the profession. Some are statutory bodies; others have wide experience and carry out teaching and/or research activities . . . It is in no sense because we fail to recognise the achievements of these bodies that we recommend that in the interests of the profession there should be one single central statutory organisation to supervise training and education and to safeguard and, when possible, to raise professional standards.'

On considering midwives it rejected the continuation of a separate statutory body but:

'At the same time we recognise the existence of real and important differences between nursing and midwifery. After careful consideration, we conclude that there are aspects of midwifery practice on which a body dealing also with all aspects of nursing could not rightly pronounce . . . We recommend therefore the setting up by statute of a Standing Midwifery Committee of the Central Nursing and Midwifery Council.'

The Committee also recommended that there should be National Boards in each of the countries of the UK to 'cover the whole field of nursing and midwifery education'.

These recommendations were incorporated into the Nurses, Midwives and Health Visitors Act 1979.

## The Nurses, Midwives and Health Visitors Act 1979

'An Act to establish a Central Council for Nursing, Midwifery and Health Visiting, and National Boards for the four parts of the United Kingdom; to make new provision with respect to the education, training, regulation and discipline of nurses, midwives and health visitors and the maintenance of a single professional register . . .'

This was one of the last Acts to pass through Parliament before the resignation of the Labour Government led by Mr Callaghan. With its passing the Central Midwives Boards for England and Wales and Scotland were dissolved as was the Joint Council in Northern Ireland and numerous other statutory and quasi-statutory bodies, and they were replaced by the United Kingdom Central Council for Nursing, Midwifery and Health Visiting (UKCC). Four National Boards were constituted with members elected by the three professions and elected members from the Boards were chosen to represent each country on the UKCC. Other places on the UKCC were taken by appointees of the Secretary of State to make the final number of members 45.

The main functions of the Council were given in section 2 of the Act:

'(1) The principal functions of the Central Council shall be to establish and improve standards of training and professional conduct for nurses, midwives and health visitors.

(2) The Council shall ensure that the standards of training they establish are such as to meet any Community obligation of the United Kingdom.

(3) The Council shall by means of rules determine the conditions of a person's being admitted to training, and the kind and standard of training to be undertaken, with a view to registration.

(4) The rules may also make provision with respect to the kind and standard of further training available to persons who are already registered.

(5) The powers of the Council shall include that of providing, in such manner as it thinks fit, advice for nurses, midwives and health visitors on standards of professional conduct.

(6) In the discharge of its functions the Council shall have proper regard for the interests of all groups within the professions, including those with minority representation.'

The National Boards were made responsible for:

- approving training courses, arranging examinations and awarding qualifications;
- approving refresher courses;
- investigating allegations of professional misconduct and referring cases when necessary to the UKCC;
- advising local supervising authorities on matters relating to the supervision of midwives; and
- receiving notification of intention to practise forms and passing this information to the UKCC.

The Act also set up Midwifery Committees at the UKCC and National Board levels and the UKCC was charged with consulting the Committee 'on all matters relating to midwifery'. Rules relating to midwifery practice were not to be approved by the Secretary of State unless they were framed in accordance with recommendations of the Council's Midwifery Committee. Similarly each Board was to consult its Committee on all matters relating to midwifery.

The Act also set up a single register divided into 'parts' for the different qualifications and trainings. These parts were not specified in the Act but it was left to the Secretary of State to determine them at a later stage. The midwifery qualification was assigned part 10. Sections 11 and 12 of the Act set out the conditions for admission to the register and removal from and restoration to the register.

Miscellaneous provisions about midwifery required the UKCC to make rules for midwifery practice including the need to give notice of intention to practise, and to attend courses of instruction. Suspension from practice and the supervision of midwifery were also included.

Section 17 of the Act states

'A person other than a registered midwife or a registered medical practitioner shall not attend a woman in childbirth.'

In 1979 the Act still banned attendance by

'a man who is a registered midwife ... except in a place approved in writing by or on behalf of the Secretary of State.'

This was later amended to allow the free practice of midwifery by men.

# The need for change

In 1988 a firm of management consultants Peat Marwick McLintock were appointed to review the statutory body structure. Their report was published in 1989. It was a very detailed report which not only looked broadly at the way the Act was functioning but examined the detailed workings of the statutory bodies. It found that the requirement for decision making to pass between National Boards and the UKCC, particularly if it were to pass through the Midwifery Committee structure, was very complex. This is best illustrated by giving a hypothetical example.

### Case study: changing practice

A midwife member of a National Board suggests that setting up an intravenous line should be accepted as part of the basic role of the midwife and incorporated into training. The Board discusses this and refers it to its Midwifery Committee, who also discuss it and recommend that it be referred to the UKCC. The UKCC then considers the issue and agrees in principle that the procedure should be incorporated into training. It consults with its Midwifery Committee who also agree. The matter is then formally referred to all the National Boards and a consensus agreement is then finally reached.

This might sound extreme, but the requirements of the Act meant that important decisions were often held up for much longer than necessary by these elaborate arrangements.

The report highlighted the seemingly unjustified structure which resulted in the body responsible for setting the standards of professional practice not being the elected body (elections were to the National Boards). It also deplored the length of time it took for cases of alleged professional misconduct to be investigated and to be heard by the UKCC Professional Conduct Committee.

The Peat Marwick McLintock report recommended fundamental changes to the primary legislation. It suggested that the UKCC should become the elected body supported by smaller, appointed National Boards with an executive function. There would be one statutory Midwifery Committee at the UKCC level.

These recommendations were accepted and amendments to the 1979 Act were incorporated into the Nurses, Midwives and Health Visitors Act 1992.

# THE CURRENT STATUTORY BODY STRUCTURE

## The UKCC

The UKCC is now the elected statutory body for nurses, midwives and health visitors. It has a maximum of sixty members, two thirds of whom are elected and one third appointed by the Secretary of State. Representation is arranged in such a way that there is a balance of both country and professional membership. Currently there are eight midwives in membership with two from each of the countries of the UK. All these midwives are on the Midwifery Committee which also has other midwife appointees, an obstetrician and another medical practitioner on it. The UKCC remains the body responsible for setting the standards required of the practitioner through the formulation of rules and codes, and for the standard, type and content of training courses. It also now has complete responsibility for all professional conduct matters at both the investigation and hearing stages.

## The National Boards

Each country still has a National Board now made up of executive and non-executive members. The executive members are also employees of the Board and the non-executive members are appointed by the relevant Secretary of State for the country. Appointments for all the statutory bodies are made in consultation with the professions. The Boards continue to be responsible for the provision of training courses by approving the courses and 'accrediting' training establishments.

# PROFESSIONAL CONDUCT

Section 8 of the Nurses, Midwives and Health Visitors Act 1992 introduced amendments to the 1979 Act. One of the functions of the previous National Boards was to investigate allegations of professional misconduct and decide whether a case should be referred to the Professional Conduct Committee of the UKCC.

All matters relating to alleged professional misconduct are now referred directly to the UKCC both for investigation and, where necessary, for a hearing.

## The Preliminary Proceedings Committee

An allegation of misconduct can arise from any source. Members of the public, colleagues, supervisors of midwives or NHS managers may all report conduct that they believe falls short of that which they would expect from the practising midwife. Additionally, cases are reported automatically by the police and the courts when a nurse or midwife has been found guilty of a criminal offence.

All cases are considered by the Preliminary Proceedings Committee. This Committee makes its decisions *in camera* (in a private meeting) and it may come to one of four decisions:

- to close the case;
- to refer the case to the Professional Conduct Committee for a hearing;
- to refer the case to a panel of professional screeners to decide whether the case should be referred to the Health Committee; or
- to close the case but issue a formal warning about future conduct.

A new power has been introduced for this Committee, the power to impose an interim suspension of registration pending early referral to the Professional Conduct Committee or Health Committee. It is difficult to assess precisely how this will be used in the future but it is intended to use the power only when there is a clear public safety issue. Any such suspension must be reviewed after three months in operation.

This new power is not such an innovation for midwives. The power to suspend from practice, which for the practitioner almost amounts to the same as an interim suspension, has always been open to the local supervising authority. The essential differences between the two mechanisms are:

- An interim suspension can apply to all nurses, midwives and health visitors on the register.
- An interim suspension applies across the UK while a suspension by a local supervising authority only applies to practice within the boundaries of that authority.
- A suspension from practice does not have to be reviewed in three months.

Again it is too early to know how suspension from practice and the interim suspension from registration will relate to each other.

## The Professional Conduct Committee

This committee is made up of members of the UKCC but when hearing a case the committee membership should have due regard to the area of practice from which the practitioner whose case is being heard comes. There is no cross-membership with the Preliminary Proceedings Committee. In the past, one of the reasons for delay in Professional Conduct Committee hearings taking place was the enormous requirements it placed upon UKCC members from minority professions like midwives. This was, of course, offset to an extent by the smaller number of cases being heard from midwifery, but delay was experienced in constituting a midwifery-focussed committee. It is now possible to add to the members of the Professional Conduct Committee from an agreed panel who are not on the parent body.

Hearings of the Professional Conduct Committee are open to the public and are held in London and at locations away from the UKCC. The proceedings are formal and the practitioner has a right to representation.

The first task of the Committee is to decide whether there has or has not been professional misconduct. If there has been no professional misconduct, the case will be closed.

If it decides there has been professional misconduct, it may then hear evidence in mitigation. This might take the form of character witnesses, reports from the midwife's employer on subsequent satisfactory practice, or reports about the work situation (staffing, workload etc.) when the misconduct took place.

The Committee then has a number of powers that it can exercise:

- it may take no further action even though misconduct has been proved;

- it may issue a formal caution which will remain on the record for five years and which may be referred to in any subsequent case of alleged misconduct occurring during that time;

- it may postpone judgment until a future time;

- it may remove the midwife's name from the register for an unspecified or a specified time;

- it may refer the case to the Panel of Screeners with a view to a Health Committee hearing; or

- it may impose an interim suspension if the hearing is adjourned.

The UKCC has produced a booklet detailing the professional conduct process and figures 2.3 and 2.4 show this. The Council also summarizes the activity of the Professional Conduct Committee in its Annual Reports.

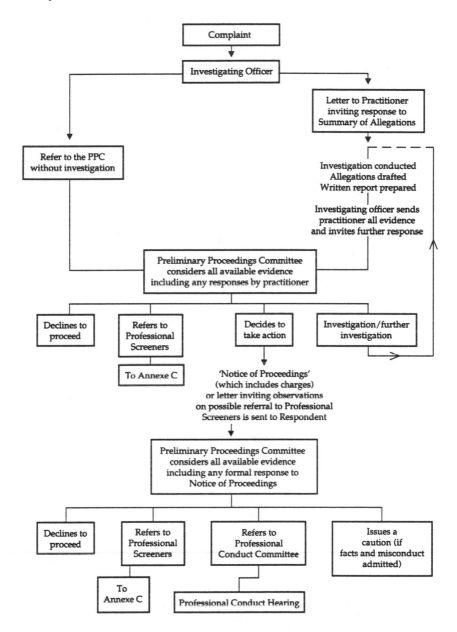

**Fig. 2.3** A simplified illustration of the process by which an allegation of misconduct is considered by the Preliminary Proceedings Committee.

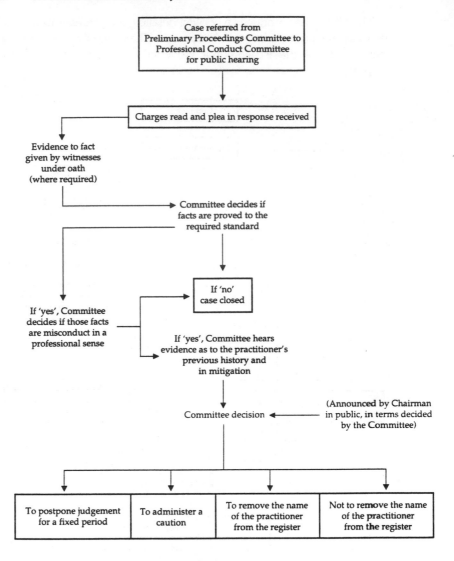

**Fig. 2.4** A simplified illustration of the process by which an allegation of misconduct is considered by the Professional Conduct Committee.

In the booklet *Complaints about Professional Conduct* [3] there is a list of offences which may lead to removal from the Register. Cases that occur frequently are:

- reckless and wilfully unskilled practice;
- concealing untoward incidents;
- failure to keep essential records;
- falsifying records;

- failure to protect or promote the interests of patients/clients;
- failure to act knowing that a colleague or subordinate is improperly treating or abusing patients;
- physical or verbal abuse of patients/clients;
- abuse of patients by improperly withholding prescribed drugs, or administering unprescribed drugs or an excess of prescribed drugs;
- theft from patients or employers;
- drug related offences;
- sexual abuse of patients; and
- breach of confidentiality.

It is usual and advisable for a midwife who finds herself at a Professional Conduct Committee hearing to be represented by her professional organization or a trade union. These organizations are skilled not only in giving formal representation on the day but in giving advice in the weeks or months leading to the hearing. If the midwife is removed from the register she may seek help from the Nurses Welfare Society which provides subsequent counselling and practical help. Chapter 5 describes in more detail what a midwife should do if she is reported to the UKCC.

## Referral to the Health Committee

Complaints about a midwife's state of health may be originated in the same way as for alleged misconduct. However cases may also be referred by the Preliminary Proceedings Committee or the Professional Conduct Committee.

When a complaint is received it is referred to a Panel of Screeners. This panel, which is made up of members of the UKCC, considers the documentary evidence and decides what medical specialist advice would be appropriate. Once the Screeners have received the medical reports they decide whether to send the case to the Health Committee. Figure 2.5 illustrates the process.

The Health Committee is made up of five members of the UKCC, meeting *in camera*. The medical examiner(s) whose reports they have will also be present. The practitioner should attend and she has the right to representation. She may also bring her own medical witnesses.

The Health Committee may:

- close the case if they consider the health impairment does not jeopardize fitness to practise;
- refer the case back to the Preliminary Proceedings Committee or the Professional Conduct Committee;
- suspend the practitioner's registration;
- remove the practitioner's name from the register;

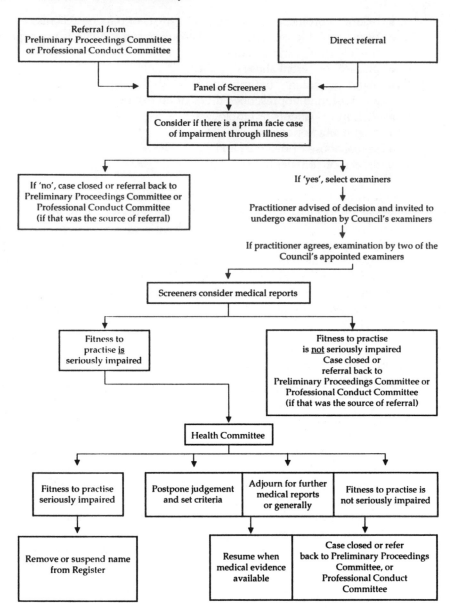

**Fig. 2.5** A simplified illustration of the process by which complaints alleging unfitness to practise are considered.

- postpone judgment; or
- impose an interim suspension if the hearing is adjourned.

## RULES AND CODES

The UKCC exercises its responsibility for the standards of practice through the formulation of statutory rules and non-statutory codes. Those that relate to the practice of the midwife are The Midwives Rules, A Midwife's Code of Practice and The Code of Professional Conduct for the Nurse, Midwife and Health Visitor.

## The Code of Professional Conduct

This Code, obtainable from the UKCC, covers the conduct expected of all the professions governed by the Council. It states that:

'Each registered nurse, midwife and health visitor shall act, at all times, and in such a manner as to:
- safeguard and promote the interests of individual patients and clients;
- serve the interests of society;
- justify public trust and confidence; and
- uphold and enhance the good standing and reputation of the professions.'

This is followed by sixteen specific requirements. As well as these, the UKCC from time to time publishes more detailed booklets which further elaborate the Code. Subjects covered include Record Keeping, Advertising and the Administration of Drugs.

## A Midwife's Code of Practice

This UKCC document is an elaboration of the standards of practice that are required of midwives under the statutory Midwives Rules. All practising midwives are issued with a personal copy whenever it is updated. As with the Code of Conduct, failure to comply can result in a charge of professional misconduct. When the Code is revised, the UKCC is guided by the Midwifery Committee and it consults with the profession on the proposed changes.

## The Midwives Rules

The 1902 Act required the Central Midwives Board to formulate rules for midwifery practice and this requirement has been continued in all subsequent legislation regarding midwifery. The Rules are formulated as secondary legislation, now forming part of the Nurses, Midwives and Health Visitors Acts 1979 and 1992. Figure 2.6 shows the frontispiece of the 1919 Rules passed by 'the Lords of His Majesty's Most Honourable Privy Council' (dated 1916). The current Rules were updated and published in November 1993.

The Rules are presented in two sections with a preceding glossary or interpretation of the terms used.

**Section A** sets out the Education Rules: entry requirements, programmes of education, the standard to be reached for admission to the Register, student indexing and examination regulations.

**Section B** gives the Practice Rules: the requirements to notify of intention to practise, to attend refresher courses, to be medically examined if necessary to prevent the spread of infection; the sphere of practice, responsibilities for administration of medicines and the

---

## AT THE COUNCIL CHAMBER, WHITEHALL,

### THE 23RD DAY OF JUNE, 1916.

### BY THE LORDS OF HIS MAJESTY'S MOST HONOURABLE

### PRIVY COUNCIL.

---

WHEREAS it is provided by Section 3 of the Midwives Act, 1902, that Rules framed by the Central Midwives Board under the said Section shall be valid only if approved by the Privy Council, and that the Privy Council before approving any such Rules shall take into consideration any representations which the General Medical Council may make with respect thereto :

And whereas the said Central Midwives Board have submitted to the Privy Council for approval certain Rules framed by them under the said Section :

NOW, THEREFORE, their Lordships, having taken into consideration the said Rules, together with a representation of the General Medical Council with respect thereto, are pleased to approve the said Rules as set forth in the Schedule hereunto annexed for the period of five years commencing on the Ist day of July next.

ALMERIC FITZROY

**Fig. 2.6** The frontispiece to the Midwives Rules 1919.

responsibility to keep records and to make practice premises available for inspection. The duties of the local supervising authority, including the power of suspension from practice and the appointment of supervisors of midwives are set also out.

## Rule 40

Undoubtedly the most important rule is rule 40, 'Responsibility and Sphere of Practice'. It is the wording of this rule that both enables the midwife's autonomy and at the same delineates its boundaries. It states

'1. A practising midwife is responsible for providing midwifery care to a mother and baby during the antenatal, intranatal and postnatal periods. In any case where there is an emergency or where she detects in the health of a mother and baby a deviation from the norm, a practising midwife shall call to her assistance a registered medical practitioner and shall forthwith report the matter to the local supervising authority.

2. A practising midwife must not, except in an emergency, undertake any treatment which she has not been trained to give either before or after registration as a midwife and which is outside her sphere of practice.'

The basis for autonomous practice lies in the first part as she only needs to refer to a registered medical practitioner when an abnormal situation occurs. Otherwise she may practise midwifery by reason of her own qualification.

This rule is very flexible in terms of what the midwife may do in her practice. It is elaborated in A Midwife's Code of Practice which discusses the requirements for competency in new skills by stating:

- that each midwife is personally responsible for maintaining and developing her competence,

- that some developments will be viewed as integral to the role of the midwife and she should be properly trained for these,

- that some developments will not be seen as integral to the midwife's role but if she is required to extend her skill to such areas of practice, it must be covered by a locally agreed policy.

Application of this interpretation of the Rules has enabled midwives to extend their practice, for example, into ultrasound scanning, ventouse extraction, and advanced family planning techniques.

### Notification of intention to practise

The Rules require that the midwife must notify each local supervising authority in which she intends to practise by the end of March each year. If, in an emergency, she practises without having given such notification she must retrospectively notify the LSA within 48 hours of having practised.

### Attendance at refresher courses

Midwives are required to attend a refresher course every five years, or, if they have not submitted an intention to practise for five years or more, must attend a course of practical and theoretical instruction for at least four weeks, the length of time to be decided by the appropriate Board. The details of this requirement are clearly described in rule 37. This rule was once very prescriptive requiring the course to be of at least five days in length and residential, although certain other studies, for example the Advanced Diploma in Midwifery, could give exemption.

There is a much greater flexibility now about what constitutes a course of instruction although whatever the midwife plans to do must still be approved by a National Board. Evidence of professional writing, of research activity, of elective professional secondment to other areas of practice may now be accepted. Any midwife contemplating a 'different' refresher course should contact one of the midwifery professional officers of the National Boards to discuss whether it may be accepted and how to apply for recognition. This should be done prospectively rather than after the experience has been undertaken to ensure that it is acceptable.

### Suspension from practice

The local supervising authority has the power to suspend a midwife from practice on two grounds. It shall do so if it is necessary to prevent the spread of infection and it may do so if the midwife is subject to any investigations by the UKCC.

In legal terms there is an interesting distinction between the words 'shall' and 'may', the first being mandatory and the second optional. It seems a strange anachronism that it remains mandatory that a midwife should be suspended from practice to protect against the spread of infection whereas a LSA has discretion in the second situation even though it may have forwarded the midwife's name to the UKCC knowing the potential outcome would be removal from the Register. Of course this flexibility protects the midwife from suspension in cases of frivolous reporting to the UKCC from members of the public but it does allow an LSA to make an indefensible decision to report a midwife for alleged misconduct and yet allow her to continue to practise.

## The administration of medicines and other forms of pain relief

As with all other areas of her practice, the Rules state that the midwife must not administer a medicine unless she has been instructed in its use. She may also only administer inhalation analgesia using apparatus approved by the UKCC.

The administration of drugs is also controlled by other legislation: the Misuse of Drugs Regulations 1985 (secondary legislation) and the Medicines Act 1971 (primary legislation) with its subsequent secondary legislation, the Medicines (Products other than Veterinary Drugs) (Prescription Only) Order 1983.

### Controlled drugs

Under the 1985 Regulations, these drugs are divided into five schedules. Midwives may obtain and use pethidine (a schedule 2 drug) and pentazocine (a schedule 3 drug) in the course of their practice.

The controlled drugs legislation requires that a strict control over supply, storage, use and destruction of these drugs is maintained. It must be possible, by referring to the records relating to these drugs, to account for the total amount issued, administered or returned and destroyed. For this to be the case in practice there are regulations specifically for midwives.

In hospital, the chief pharmacist is responsible for the hospital stocks. All drugs issued to wards must be properly requisitioned. The ward sister is responsible for the maintenance of drugs records and controlled drugs should be kept in a locked compartment of a fixed locked cupboard. The numbers of drugs administered should tally with the remaining stock which should be regularly checked. Controlled drugs may be administered by midwives using the system of doctors' standing orders. The drugs on the list will be subject to local agreement. It is the responsibility of the pharmacist to destroy out-of-date stock. The midwife should return such stock to the pharmacy.

There are different arrangements for the midwife working in the community.

Such a midwife must obtain her controlled drugs using a supply order form authorized by the supervisor of midwives. She must then obtain the drugs from a pharmacy with whom she has a previous arrangement. This may be the local hospital pharmacy. She must keep her own personal register of drugs into which she must record the details of supply, administration, return or destruction of drugs. This register must be made available for inspection by the supervisor of midwives when required. She must store the drugs in a fixed, locked cupboard accessible only to her.

The midwife may only destroy controlled drugs in the presence of an authorized person, who may be:

- a supervisor of midwives in England, Wales and Northern Ireland,
- a Regional Pharmaceutical Officer in England,
- the Pharmaceutical Adviser, Welsh Office,
- the Chief Administrative Pharmaceutical Officer of the Health Boards in Scotland
- an inspector appointed by the Northern Ireland Department of Health and Social Services
- medical officers of the Regional Medical Services in England, Scotland and Wales,
- an inspector of the Pharmaceutical Society of Great Britain,
- a police officer, or
- an inspector of the Home Office Drugs Branch.

Of course in some cases it is the supervisor of midwives who would oversee the destruction of these drugs, but the most common practice is for the midwife to exchange her out-of-date stock at a designated pharmacy and the pharmacy then arranges for destruction of its stocks.

### Prescription only medicines
Midwives may use a limited list of these drugs in the course of their practice. They include analgesics, drugs for the control of postpartum haemorrhage, sedatives and drugs for neonatal resuscitation.

### Licensed/unlicensed drugs
All the drugs that a midwife may give have to be licensed for use in the UK. This includes intramuscular vitamin K. A study in the early 1990s indicated a possible link with this and childhood cancer and use of the intravenous route was stopped. However, there was no licensed oral preparation and advice from the Department of Health in 1993 was that the oral preparation should be individually prescribed by a doctor prior to administration.

## Miscellaneous legislative requirements

### The Births and Deaths Registration Acts and Public Health Acts

Under these Acts the midwife is required to do two things:

Firstly, to notify a birth, whether liveborn or stillborn, to the appropriate medical officer within 36 hours of the birth. This is not exclusively the responsibility of the midwife, but of anyone who attends the birth. In practice it is almost always the midwife who does this.

Secondly, she is required to register a birth within 42 days (in Scotland 21 days) of the birth if the parents fail to do so. In practice this is very rarely ever done by the midwife as the Registrar of Births will make every effort to get the parents to register their baby. In the case of their default, however, the midwife present at the delivery may be approached to do so. For the child, registration is essential as it is the process that results in recognition of the child for all subsequent administrative purposes.

### Certification of a stillbirth

The midwife should make every effort to obtain medical certification of a stillbirth. A doctor present at the delivery or who has attended the woman during pregnancy and has subsequently examined the body will in most circumstances issue the certificate. If this is impossible to arrange, the midwife may complete the certificate if she was present at the delivery or examined the body.

### Jury service

Under the various Juries Acts, midwives are exempt from serving on a jury.

## CONTROVERSIES SURROUNDING STATUTORY CONTROL

Merger of the three professions into one statutory framework in 1979 was not without its critics. Some of the gravest reservations were expressed by midwives who valued the separate nature of the Midwives Acts. When the 1979 Act was passed it was hoped that the proper use of the Midwifery Committees would preserve the separate identity of midwifery.

In 1990 the English National Board, followed by the Welsh National Board, decided to restructure its professional and education advisory staff, introducing for each of them a more generic role. The Midwifery Committee at the English National Board disagreed with this redefinition of roles as not being in the best interests of midwifery. This recommendation was rejected by the full Board. The objections to this led to the setting up of a pressure group, the Midwives Legislation Group, which has the aim of restoring separate legislation for midwives.

### The case for professional legislation

The arguments for a restoration of a Midwives Act seem clear. Midwifery, because of the disparity in numbers, will always be 'out-voted' by the nursing profession, potentially resulting in an erosion of the autonomous position of the midwife. All other professions enjoy their own legislation and indeed a fundamental definition of a separate profession is that it controls its own affairs, its standards of practice, entry into its education system, standards of training and maintenance of its own register. If compromises were theoretically made in 1979, they seemed palpably apparent when the decisions of the Midwifery Committees could so easily be ignored.

The Midwives Legislation Group has received legal advice on the wording of new legislation and has been actively seeking support from the profession. The branch delegates' meeting of the 1990 Annual Conference of the Royal College of Midwives voted to support a campaign for new legislation, although the Council of the College decided first to set up a commission to examine all the implications of the present legislation. This commission, chaired by Lady Wyndham Kaye, concluded that there was insufficient evidence that the legislation was working against the interests of midwifery but that this could change in the future. The College set up a group – Legislation Watch – which would monitor the statutory position of midwifery.

## The case against professional legislation

There are equally persuasive arguments against pursuing separate legislation, particularly at present.

The usual view of a profession is a group of people bound together by an agreed standard of conduct, agreed rules of admission to the profession and bound by the knowledge generated by its members. The group is accepted as acting altruistically in the best interests of the public and that any regulations, statutory or otherwise, are designed to protect the public. Hence the first words in the UKCC Code of Professional Conduct for the Nurse, Midwife and Health Visitor are:

'Each registered nurse, midwife and health visitor shall act, at all times, in such a manner as to:
- safeguard and promote the interests of individual patients and clients;
- serve the interests of society;
- justify public trust and confidence; and
- uphold and enhance the good standing and reputation of the profession.'

There is an alternative, and much more negative, view of the professions and thus of their statutory regulation. Everett Hughes [4] claimed that the professions act as powerful ideological monopolies which define the needs of the consumer, the manner of the service and the way society views their activities.

'Not merely do the practitioners, by virtue of gaining admission to the charmed circle of colleagues, individually exercise the licence to do things others do not, but collectively they presume to tell society what is good and right for the individual and for society at large in some aspect of life. Indeed they set the very terms in which people may think about this aspect of life.'

In short the profession and the regulatory mechanisms related to it function not for the protection of the public, but for the protection of the profession.

Taken to its logical conclusion, this view of professional regulation contradicts the traditional midwifery concept of being with women, and, if statutory regulation implicitly protects the professional from the outside world, it may also implicitly place barriers between the midwife and the women she should be caring for.

Enforcement of section 17 of the 1979 Act would do just that. Any midwife would be justified in reporting an infringement of that section (for example a husband planning to deliver his wife) to the LSA, and any LSA would be justified in pursuing the case in the courts. It has happened. But what would such action achieve? It certainly would not engender future trust between the couple and midwives. They might even be tempted to 'go underground' when the next pregnancy occurs.

A second argument for introducing some caution into the pursuit of legislation for its own sake is the damaging effect it can have in limiting justifiable human activity.

The history of midwifery legislation and legal licensure demonstrates this. De Vries [5] in his examination of the effect of regulation on midwifery states:

'Most physicians opposed the registration of midwives on the grounds that legal recognition would enhance the midwife's position, take births away from doctors and hinder the development of obstetrics . . . On the other hand, and for many of the same reasons, midwives were often anxious to see some type of licensing law passed, viewing such legislation as a necessary condition for survival. On the surface these positions seem consistent with the best interests of the occupations involved, but as the outcomes of midwife regulation are investigated, this assumption becomes questionable. Contrary to the beliefs of both doctors and midwives, these regulatory acts did not result in the establishment of an independent profession of midwifery, but rather placed the midwife in a position where her autonomy has steadily declined.'

Oakley and Houd (1990) put the argument succinctly.

'Licensing has a double message: to recognise the value of what midwives do and to limit what in the future they will be able to do.' [6]

Nowhere is this message more powerfully seen than in the UK with arguably one of the most stable regulatory mechanisms in the world, but one which requires every midwife to notify that she intends to practise on an annual basis. Good for statistics maybe, but what other profession is controlled in this way? What other profession has a set of Rules that *prescribe in law* the need to keep records and to open practice premises for inspection, and a duty to be medically examined and to be supervised? What other profession has had to wait 70 years before it achieved chairmanship of its own regulating body? It was 1973 before a midwife became the Chairman of the Central Midwives Board. And, true to the De Vries argument, this separate regulating body presided over a gradual decline in the autonomous position of the midwife.

This leads to the third and potentially most powerful argument against pursuing legislation at least for the time being; that the fortunes of occupational groups, whether professions or otherwise, depend more on what they do and are seen to be doing than on whether they have legislative protection.

The nadir of the UK midwifery profession was probably reached in the mid-1970s after a slow half century attrition of its status. Some believed that the midwife had followed her American sisters into obstetric nursing. The Central Midwives Board 'presided' over this decline. Indeed when it was at its most rapid, in the 1970s, was the time when the Board was at last controlled by midwives. Yet the recent resurgence of midwifery has occurred during the time when the UKCC has been the regulating body.

There seems to be no relationship between the form of midwifery regulation and the autonomy of the profession. Rather it would seem that it is what midwives do that is the deciding factor in whether they work autonomously or not. Demonstration of the needs of women for midwifery care and demonstration by midwives that they can offer that expert, knowledgeable and responsive care is a much more powerful incentive for society to recognize the worth of midwifery than legislative protection.

The anarchist might argue that all regulatory legislation should be repealed. Others may be much more cautious, arguing that the effect of having no legal regulatory mechanism may put women at risk. Whatever the long term solution, any future legislation should be framed in such a way that it offers protection to women without restricting the midwife in the proper pursuit of her trade.

## SUMMARY

Midwifery is a profession regulated by statutory controls. The usual reasons given for this are protection of the public and protection of the profession.

Statutory regulation includes the setting of standards for practice and education, and the maintenance of a professional register.

An alternative view interprets the legislation of the twentieth century as an attempt to control the activities of the midwife.

## FURTHER ACTION

- Contact the UKCC to arrange to attend an open meeting of the Council.

- Invite the Midwifery Officer at the UKCC to give a talk about the functions of the Council and her role in particular.

- Talk to a midwifery officer at your National Board to see if you can visit the Board offices to find out how they function.

## REFERENCES

1. Royal College of Midwives. *Behind the Blue Door*. London, RCM, 1981.
2. Department of Health and Social Services. *Report of the Committee on Nursing* (Chairman: Asa Briggs). London, HMSO, 1972.
3. United Kingdom Central Council for Nursing, Midwifery and Health Visiting. *Complaints about Professional Conduct*. London, UKCC, 1993.
4. Hughes, Everett Cherrington. *Men and their Work*. Glencoe, Ill., The Free Press, 1958.
5. De Vries, R.G. *Midwifery and the Problem of Licensure. Research in the Sociology of Health Care 2*. Greenwich, Conn., Jai Press Inc. 1982.
6. Oakley, A. and Houd, S. *Helpers in Childbirth: midwifery today*. Hemisphere Publishing on behalf of the WHO regional Office for Europe, 1990.

# Chapter 3
# The Supervision of Midwives

## AN HISTORICAL OVERVIEW

### The Midwives Act 1902

Midwifery is unique amongst the professions for having a local mechanism to enforce the statutory regulation of its activity. The principle of the supervision of midwives was incorporated into the Midwives Act 1902. This Act required the designation of local supervising authorities (then the Borough Councils) and gave them statutory powers:

(1) to exercise general supervision over all midwives practising within their area in accordance with the rules to be laid down under the Act;

(2) to investigate charges of malpractice, negligence or misconduct on the part of any midwife practising within their area and, should a *prima facie* case be established, to report the same to the Central Midwives Board (CMB);

(3) to suspend any midwife from practice, in accordance with the rules under the Act, if such suspension appeared necessary in order to prevent the spread of infection;

(4) to report at once to the CMB the name of any midwife practising in their area convicted of an offence;

(5) during the month of January of each year to supply the secretary of the CMB with the names and addresses of all midwives who, during the preceding year, have notified their intention to practise within their area, and to keep a current copy of the Roll of Midwives accessible at all reasonable times for public inspection;

(6) to report to the CMB the death of any midwife or any change in the name or address of any midwife in their area so that the necessary alteration may be made to the Roll.

(7) to give due notice of the effect of the Act so far as practicable to persons at present using the title of midwife.

The original Act did not mention the Supervisor of Midwives, but the LSAs were given the power to delegate any of the powers conferred or imposed on them to a committee on which, it was stated, women might sit!

Over the years the process of delegation developed into delegation to one person rather than to a committee, proof, perhaps, that committees might be very good at discussion but not efficient at doing things! However, it would seem that it was common practice to give responsibility for the supervision of midwives to a health visitor. Further, regulations delineating the process for the supervision of midwives were introduced in section 2 of the Midwives Act 1936 and in 1937 a letter was sent from the Ministry of Health to the LSAs elaborating on the revised requirements for supervision.

## The Ministry of Health letter

This letter is fundamental to the understanding of both the development of supervision and to some of the claims for its functions today and the text is given in full.

'Sir

(1) I am directed by the Minister of Health to enclose for the information of the Council copies of the Regulations which he has made under Section 9(2) of the Midwives Act 1936, prescribing the qualifications of persons appointed by Local Supervising Authorities under Section 8 of the Midwives Act, 1902, to exercise supervision over midwives practising in their areas. The Regulations, which have been made after consultation with the Central Midwives Board and the Association of Local Authorities concerned, will come into operation on the 1st June next.

(2) It will be observed that the Regulations apply to persons appointed as Supervisors of Midwives on or after that date, but in view of the importance of entrusting this work to persons with the necessary qualifications and experience, the Minister suggests that each Authority should review their arrangements for the supervision of midwives and should take the earliest opportunity for effecting any changes which may be desirable having regard to the qualifications prescribed by the Regulations. This is of particular importance at the present time when the new service of salaried midwives under the Act of 1936 is about to be established throughout the country.

(3) The Departmental Committee on Midwives, which reported in 1929, pointed out that the inspection of midwives by a person

without adequate experience of practical midwifery has a bad psychological effect upon the midwife, and reacts unfavourably on her methods of practice, as she is deprived of the opportunity for guidance on professional matters affecting the well-being of her patients which she would receive from a properly qualified inspector. In particular, the Committee strongly deprecated the employment as inspectors of midwives of Health Visitors with little or no practical experience of midwifery. The Minister endorses these views, and it will be seen that the Regulations require that persons appointed in future to supervise midwives shall have had adequate experience in the practice of midwifery.

(4) The Departmental Committee also drew attention to the fact that an inspector of midwives should be regarded as the counsellor and friend of the midwives, rather than a relentless critic, and should be one who is ready to instruct the midwives in the various points of difficulty which arise from time to time in connection with their work and make them feel that there is always someone to whom they can look for sympathetic understanding of the laborious nature of their profession. The Minister feels that it is scarcely necessary for him to emphasise the importance of appointing persons who not only possess the necessary professional qualifications, but who also have the essential qualities of sympathy and tact, and he thinks it desirable that the title of 'Inspector of Midwives' should be superseded by that of 'Supervisor of Midwives' which is that used in the Regulations.

(5) The Regulations prescribe qualifications for a Medical Supervisor, and a non-Medical Supervisor, respectively, and it is within the discretion of each Authority to appoint either one or the other, or both. But in large areas it appears to the Minister that the most desirable arrangement would generally be to appoint a Medical Supervisor, acting under the direction of the Medical Officer of Health, to exercise general supervision over the midwives practising in the area, and non-Medical Supervisors to work under the instructions of the Medical Supervisor and perform the routine duties of supervision.

(6) The Minister appreciates that at the outset it may be difficult in some cases to secure Medical Supervisors who possess all the qualifications prescribed in Article 3 of the Regulations, and if necessary he will be prepared to consider the question of using the dispensing power which is contained in Article 5. He thinks it desirable, however, to point out that the words "some branch of obstetric work" in Article 3 have a wide range, and include the conduct of ante-natal clinics, the duties of administrative officers

in a maternity department, the investigation or treatment of puerperal fever, obstetric research, etc.

(7) In conclusion, the Minister wishes to emphasise the fact that the duties of a Supervisor of Midwives extend to all the midwives practising in the area of the Authority, and that a distinction should be drawn between an officer holding this post and one who is appointed as a Superintendent or Senior Midwife to control the work of the salaried midwives appointed by the Authority. The Minister is advised that it is not desirable for a Supervisor of Midwives to be engaged in the actual practice of midwifery.

(8) A copy of this circular has been sent to the Medical Officer of Health.

> I am, Sir,
> Your obedient Servant,
>
> Assistant Secretary.'

The principles of this letter continued to be applied until the 1970s and some of them still apply today. The 1991 Code of Practice paragraph 3.7.5. states:

'The supervisor of midwives' role as a supportive colleague, counsellor and advisor should be developed in order to promote a positive working relationship which is conducive to maintaining and improving standards of care.'

## Subsequent developments

Although there was a major consolidation of midwifery legislation in 1951, the statutory requirements for the supervision of midwives were largely unchanged. In fact the first significant alteration to the legislation came about as the result of pressures external to the profession.

In 1974 the NHS experienced the first re-organization since its inception. The tripartite system of administration which effectively separated the hospital, community and contracted services (general practice, dentistry, etc.) was dissolved and all services were brought together under unified authorities. District midwives, who were still employed by the local authorities, became employees of the new health authorities. Amendments to the legislation were introduced to make Regional Health Authorities (England), Area Health Authorities (Wales), Health Boards (Scotland) and Health and Social Services Boards (Northern Ireland) the local supervising authorities.

In 1977 a further amendment abolished the requirement for a

medical supervisor of midwives. Midwives were at last, after 75 years, deemed capable of supervising themselves.

Statutory changes to the system since then have concentrated on the training and up-dating of the supervisor, introducing required attendance at an induction course on first being appointed and afterwards, at intervals, at specially designed refresher courses.

# THE PRESENT ARRANGEMENTS

The current statutory requirements for supervision are contained in the Nurses, Midwives and Health Visitors Act 1979 and in rules 44 and 45 of the Midwives Rules.

## Qualification and administrative requirements

To be a supervisor of midwives a person shall be a registered midwife with either:

- three years practising experience, one of which should be within two years of appointment, or
- further experience as required by the UKCC.

She shall have had a course of instruction within the three years preceding her appointment and should attend further approved courses at intervals of five years.

Rule 45 requires that each LSA shall publish

(1) the date in March by which the intention to practise notices should be received and by whom;
(2) the way it will investigate cases of alleged misconduct; and
(3) how it will decide upon suspension from practice.

It is also required to publish

(1) the list of its supervisors;
(2) details of how midwives will have continuous access to a supervisor of midwives; and
(3) how it will exercise supervision.

The LSAs remain as they were in 1974, except that the Area Health Authorities in Wales have changed their title to District Health Authority.

There have however been distinct developments in the organization of supervision unrelated to the statutory position.

## Who the supervisors are

The 1937 letter indicated that the supervisor should not be drawn either from midwifery management or current practitioners, but this is now the rule rather than the exception. Since the development of midwifery management during the early part of the 1970s supervision has increasingly been linked to senior midwifery management posts. Recently more supervisors have been appointed from the clinical management levels, such as clinical team leaders and delivery suite clinical managers, modifying the original suggestion in 1937 that the midwife should not be in direct clinical practice.

## What supervisors do

All LSAs are required by the Midwives Rules to publish in writing 'details of how the practice of midwives will be supervised'. These documents vary from authority to authority but there is a core of work that is common to all. Supervisors are required to:

- be responsible for collection and collation of the midwives' intention to practise notices;

- conduct regular supervisory visits to each midwife to review her standard of practice, audit her drugs records and general record keeping and inspect her practice premises where necessary;

- advise the LSA in situations where there may be professional misconduct and where suspension from practice and referral to the UKCC is being considered;

- assess the training needs of the midwives she supervises, identify new skills for which training is required, facilitate any such training, and ensure that all midwives have the opportunity to meet the requirements for refresher courses;

- provide supply order forms for the supply of pethidine, and act as an authorized person for the destruction of controlled drugs (this is rarely required);

- be available to the midwives she supervises to discuss practice issues (the Code of Practice particularly highlights the need for the supervisor to be available if a midwife fails to obtain medical support for a home confinement or where the parents refuse medical cover);

- receive notifications of maternal death, stillbirth or neonatal death from midwives and, where necessary, investigate the circumstances of the death; and

- arrange for the medical examination of a midwife if it is thought necessary to prevent the spread of infection.

Although these requirements seem straightforward, the problems that a supervisor faces can be complex. She may also be a manager and her managerial and supervisory duties are often linked. The solutions are not always apparent as the following case study shows.

## Case study: keeping records

### The background

Margaret is a community midwife. She has been in her job for over ten years. Her LSA requires the supervisors to visit each midwife annually to check the requirements of the Midwives Rules are being met. The last visit to Margaret was satisfactory and there has been nothing within the year to suggest that she was not carrying out her duties properly.

An important part of the visit is to audit the record keeping of the midwife. On the next occasion, Catherine, the supervisor, finds Margaret's records unsatisfactory. They are not properly filed so that retrieval is difficult, but, more importantly, there are omissions. Very few of the postnatal notes have been completed although, according to work sheets and the records of the unit, Margaret regularly took one or two transfers evey day.

There was also evidence that she had not been doing antenatal home visits despite an authority policy which required that each woman would have at least one visit.

### The strict approach

Margaret has breached the Midwives Rules as well as the authority policies. Failure to meet the record keeping requirements of the Rules is a *prima facie* case of misconduct. For this, one course of action for the supervisor would be to report it to the LSA and the LSA, after consideration, might report Margaret to the UKCC.

The supervisor is Margaret's manager. She is also concerned that Margaret has not followed her employer's policy requirements. The supervisor acting as manager therefore could have decided that she should take appropriate disciplinary action. She could have suspended Margaret from duty while an investigation took place. She could also have reported her to the LSA which could have suspended Margaret from practice while her name was forwarded to the UKCC.

This is a fairly typical situation and one that demonstrates clearly the close association between supervision and management. Acting in this way, however, the supervisor could certainly not be seen as counsellor and friend nor would it necessarily be good management.

### The pragmatic approach

Margaret's work had been entirely satisfactory until the year preceding Catherine's visit. Instead of taking immediate action against Margaret,

Catherine decided first to investigate Margaret's situation informally. She decided to find out whether there was a reason for the deterioration in practice. She asked Margaret if she had any problems. At first Margaret denied any difficulties. Then, understanding that she was facing disciplinary action she told Catherine of the problems she had been having.

Her son in his early twenties had been working about ten miles away from home. It was the first job he had had since leaving school at sixteen and being unemployed for three years. On his way home one night he was stopped by the police and breathalysed. He lost his driving licence and, because of poor public transport, could not get to work. Margaret did not tell anyone about this but began taking her son to and from work whilst at the same time continuing to carry out her extensive case load.

Knowing this Catherine took a very different approach. She remembered what her statutory role really was – to ensure that the statutory requirements are met so that the public is protected from the bad practitioner. Margaret was clearly not a bad practitioner, just a woman with personal problems. Reporting her case to the UKCC would not solve the difficulty and the employer could lose an otherwise good midwife.

The supervisor decided to take disciplinary action only, and Margaret was eventually given a first written warning. This generated a formal record in her personal file. Margaret, with the help of her professional organization's representative, discussed with the supervisor/manager how she might alleviate the situation for herself. It was decided that she would work for a year on a part-time basis and then be restored to full-time work. She was also very relieved that her colleagues now knew about her problems and understood them. Finally, the supervisor discussed Margaret's training needs with her and made arrangements for Margaret to attend a course on legal issues in midwifery in which there was a major component on the importance of record keeping.

With this flexible approach, and an appropriate combination of management and supervision, Margaret returned to her full duties one year later. Her son found a flat in the town where he worked.

### Other possibilities

Before leaving this case, there might have been another reason for Margaret's poor practice; she may have been ill herself. It might have been a physical or mental illness or she might have started drinking heavily. In this case in her manager's role Catherine should consider referral to occupational health whereas in her supervisor's role she should consider referral to the Health Committee of the UKCC. She might also assess that Margaret could continue to be a risk to her clients. As a manager, she might suspend Margaret from duty; as a supervisor she might report Margaret to the LSA who would consider referral to the Health Committee.

Generally, as this case illustrates, a flexible approach by a supervisor leads to a much more satisfactory outcome. It is clear that the work can be difficult and requires a range of skills that are not always recognized by the practising midwife.

# DOES SUPERVISION WORK?

## The problem

Until the mid 1980s there appeared to be little interest in the process of midwifery supervision. A literature search on the topic conducted in 1985 drew a blank – there was apparently no published material at the time. Midwifery text books were the only source of information and they merely reiterated the legislative requirements. There was some empirical evidence at the time, from a workshop held by the English National Board in 1983, that there were some difficulties in defining the role.

This workshop was designed to examine the current legislation, to look at the organizational structure for midwifery, to clarify the role of the supervisor and to identify the difference between the role of the supervisor and the role of the manager. One of the conclusions of the unpublished report of its findings (R. Jenkins, unpublished observations) was that supervisors needed to be given a clear understanding of the difference between supervision and management. Thirty years before, the Ministry of Health letter also anticipated the difficulty of separating the two roles and suggested that they should not be combined into one midwife's work.

In 1985 Hughes [1] stated that

'confusion between managerial and supervisory roles has on occasion led to managers telling a midwife that she was suspended from practice when the manager, not being a recognised supervisor, had no right to do this.'

Even this claim failed to understand that the supervisor has no right to suspend a midwife from practice. This responsibility lies with the LSA.

In 1986 a report in *The Guardian* quoted a letter from the Chairman of the Northern Regional Health Authority:

'there are already examples of personnel officers being involved in discussion about midwifery practice and threatening disciplinary action without understanding the discipline which exists with the supervisory regulations for midwifery.' [2]

The relationship between the supervisor and the midwives she supervises has also been questioned. There was clearly a problem in 1937 which led the Minister to describe her role as 'counsellor and friend' rather than 'relentless critic'. Isherwood [3] asks 'Would a midwife who is worried and insecure about her practice, or who is concerned about staffing levels find it easy to approach such a person?' She suggests that the demands on the supervisor of being both a supporter but the potential 'professional discipliner' must inevitably lead to role conflict.

## The origins of the problem

Statutory professional supervision is unique to midwifery so it is not possible to compare the experience in the profession with any other professional group. It is impossible therefore to say whether the problems are unique to midwifery or unique to supervision. It is however possible to trace some of the possible antecedents to the uneasy position of supervision today.

The overt reason for local statutory supervision in 1902 was to ensure that the national statutory regulations would be complied with by a profession that was largely self-employed. Chapter 2 discussed the possibility that legislation can be used to control and this argument can also be put in relation to supervision. Again, looking at the Regulations of 1937, the system was further strengthened with the introduction of the medical and non-medical supervisors. One interpretation of the Regulations is that they strengthened the position of the midwife *vis à vis* the health visitor. It is possible, however, to interpret them as a gender issue. The Medical Officer would undoubtedly have been a man in 1937 whereas the non-medical supervisor would have been a woman. The Regulations introduced a familiar gender construct: the masculine role one of leadership, decision making and with greater remuneration; the female role one of subordination, lower pay and yet the one expected to do the work.

If there was always a covert function of supervision onto which overt change was from time to time superimposed, it would not be surprising if the result was role ambiguity. In 1977 the position of medical supervisor was abolished, leaving supervision to the midwifery profession so that any underlying gender problems were resolved, but others remain.

There have been other more explicit changes which may have served to make the traditional provision of supervision seem anachronistic. Communications were poor at the beginning of the century and the rigour of an employer/employee contract could not be used to enforce standards from a central office in London. Supervision was the mechanism introduced to ensure compliance with the statutory regulations amongst a self-employed group who were often isolated.

All this has changed. Midwives are for the most part employees; communication systems are rapid and very powerful; most midwives work in large and controlled establishments (hospitals) and those who work in the community are usually managed from the hospital base. Yet there has been almost no change in the statutory requirements. Even the advice in the 1937 letter, that combining management and supervision may create problems, has largely been ignored.

Finally the environment within which supervision operates has changed. When first introduced supervision was a local authority responsibility. These authorities were fairly small and most had few supervisors. The organizational link between the supervisor and the LSA was very close. In 1974, when health care was unified, in England the Regional Health Authorities became the LSAs. This was in a very hierarchical NHS and an equally hierarchical nursing and midwifery managerial structure. Statutory supervision however remained a flattened structure and this has created further problems.

Within the supervisor network itself there were midwives at every level of the managerial hierarchy whereas they were in law considered equal for supervision purposes. With one hat on, an equal; with another, a subordinate. Secondly, some of the supervisors in first-line management positions were so far removed managerially from the regional level that they had difficulty in having any substantial contact. The official voice of supervision at regional level was the Regional Nursing Officer, who was usually a nurse. Although there have been some notable exceptions, there was no reason why these nurses should be committed to midwifery supervision, particularly as many of them saw the divisions that existed within midwifery itself over the role.

The original overt and covert reasons for supervision have gone and the structure within which it is supposed to function has changed, yet there has been little legislative will to alter its statutory basis. It is not surprising that the debate on the role of the supervisor has continued even though there have been some moves to adapt its structure even if not the legal framework.

## Changes to supervision

There have been some attempts to improve the functioning of supervision. The English National Board workshop referred to above recommended that all new supervisors should attend an introductory course, and this was implemented soon afterwards. Supervisors now are also required to attend specially focussed refresher courses every five years.

There have also been changes to the structural pattern of supervision. The 1983 workshop considered two structures. In law all supervisors have equal status and equal access to the LSA. Figure 3.1 shows the flattened nature of statutory supervision whereas figure 3.2 shows a suggested hierarchical structure.

At the time the workshop rejected the introduction of any change to the relationship between supervisors. A small unpublished study into role conflict among supervisors in Wales in 1985 (R. Jenkins, unpublished observations) revealed however that some authorities were

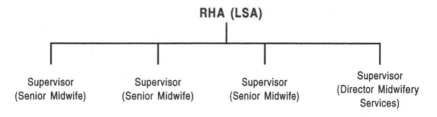

**Fig. 3.1** A flattened structure for midwifery supervision.

operating supervision in a hierarchical way. The study also showed that role conflict existed. When other factors where examined there was no correlation between length of supervision experience and role conflict but a weak association was found between the operation of supervision as a hierarchy and a reduction in role conflict.

Supervision of midwifery has now adopted hierarchical structures. LSAs now operate supervisors' networks and encourage regular contact between their supervisors. One supervisor, usually one of the most senior of the midwife managers but occasionally a midwife employed at region level, acts as a link supervisor, thus not taking a recognized superior role but nevertheless acting in a leadership capacity.

Present evidence would suggest that problems still exist. Interestingly some of the most outspoken of the critics come from the independent sector. This sector most resembles midwifery organization when the 1902 Act was passed. They are, however, more vulnerable if they are suspended from practice by an LSA. Unlike the NHS midwife, the independent midwife loses her income on suspension.

Another real cause for concern is the number of supervisors of midwives to whom an independent midwife has to relate. Because the legal requirement is to notify intention to practise to every LSA where she works, the midwife who works across multiple LSAs, will need to make multiple supervisor contacts.

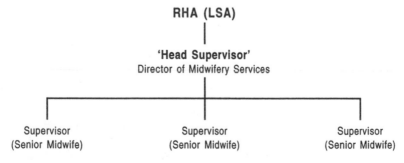

**Fig. 3.2** A hierarchical structure for midwifery supervision.

# THE FUTURE OF SUPERVISION

Supervision faces two potential futures, one which will happen as a result of proposed changes to the NHS and one that may happen, and whether it does will ultimately depend on the views of the profession.

## Anticipated NHS changes

In November 1993 the Secretary of State announced proposed changes to the health service management in England. In April 1994 the fourteen Regional Health Authorities (RHAs) were reduced to eight by a process of amalgamation. In April 1995 legislation will be introduced that will abolish the statutory nature of the RHA. Concurrent with this, there is to be an increase in the outposted offices of the NHS Executive so that there is one in each of the geographical areas of the RHAs. No-one expects the RHAs to survive even though they are not being officially abolished. The statutory RHAs are also the local supervising authorities. There are two possible bodies which could be given responsibility for supervision, the NHS Executive outposts or the purchasing authorities, either District Health Authorities or the newer amalgamated purchasers or commissioning bodies.

If the NHS Executive outposts become the LSAs, links between the UKCC and the LSAs will continue to be easy. There will be just eight offices and eight responsible officers to communicate with. Supervision will retain its current profile to a large extent. Placing supervision at this level will result in a large area of responsibility which might be large enough to justify the appointment of a midwife.

The disadvantages of supervision being placed with the NHS Executive reflect some of its historical problems. First the Executive is part of the clear management chain in the NHS, whereas the RHAs were always outside pure line management, acting in an overseeing and monitoring capacity. Placing supervision with the Executive may exacerbate the problems of role conflict between management and supervision responsibilities. Secondly, the larger NHS Executive offices are likely to be even more remote from the day-to-day operation of supervision than the RHAs.

The alternative placement for supervision, the District Health Authority, would bring supervision to a level closer to midwifery practice and return therefore to a situation that more nearly resembles the pre-1974 era. These District Health Authorities are operating outside the line management mechanisms as their functions are now related to health care purchase. The relationship with the UKCC will, however, be more complex as there will many more personnel to relate to. At this level of responsibility it will be unlikely to attract a full-time post. However in responding to their other requirements to assess the health care needs of their populations, some health authorities are employing midwives to work on midwifery and related women's health issues along with supervision.

## Other possible developments

There is another possible future role for supervision in the future organization and delivery of health care. The 1989 White Paper, *Working for Patients*, introduced Government interest in spreading the practice of medical audit, defined as

> 'a systematic, critical analysis of the quality of medical care including the procedures used for diagnosis and treatment, the use of resources, and the resulting outcome for the patient.' [4]

At the time the policy emphasis was on medical audit, as was the funding to support it.

There has been a change in view and a publication from the Department of Health calls for clinical, multidisciplinary audit to be supported. [5] Auditing care is not a statutory function even though it was discussed in a White Paper; rather the Government has made it clear that it regards audit as a professional matter.

The supervisor of midwives, with her traditional role of upholding the standards of practice of the midwives in her area could co-ordinate the audit of midwifery practice and be responsible for representing this into the multidisciplinary audit activity.

## Has supervision a future?

For all its apparent faults and the criticisms levelled at it, supervision has many defenders within the profession. Lansdell states

> 'The statutory system of supervision . . . should not be undervalued. It is to be hoped that few midwives these days would regard their supervisor of midwives as a relentless critic, but many could benefit by making fuller use of her as counsellor and friend in the increasingly demanding work they undertake.' [6]

But this leaves unanswered some important questions. What proven benefit is supervision to outcomes of maternity care? Why should midwifery be the only profession to be subjected to this form of control? If there are benefits or potential benefits to such a system of professional regulation, should it not be extended to all?

The Department of Health report, *Assessing the Effects of Health Technologies*, defines these technologies as including 'all the methods used by health professionals to promote health, to prevent disease, and to improve rehabilitation and long-term care. These methods include "hardware" such as syringes, medicines and high technology diagnostic imaging equipment; "software" such as health education, diagnostic and therapeutic policies; as well as the skills and time of people working in the health services.' [7]

Supervision costs money.

- There is an opportunity cost, as time taken in supervision activities could be used for clinical, managerial or education work.
- The initial preparation of the supervisor and subsequent refresher courses are an additional cost.
- The regional co-ordination of supervision requires meeting time and support.

There has been no rigorous examination of its value to standards of clinical care, especially now that other forms of management audit and legal control may be more effective. Many medical technologies are now facing criticism for lack of assessment, and the same can apply to supervision.

However, unlike many of the technologies, which have become such integral parts of clinical care that it is now difficult to set up relevant research, it should be possible to perform observational research into midwifery supervision. There are enough safeguards in the health care system to suspend supervision in one or two regions and then study the effect of this upon maternity care outcomes.

Such a study might answer one of the other questions on supervision; should it be extended to other professions? If a statutory mechanism can be shown to make a difference in the adoption, development and maintenance of professional standards, then should it perhaps be considered for the general practitioner, the hospital consultant, the dentist and others?

The debate so far has been on the appropriateness of midwifery supervision as a mechanism for ensuring professional standards. The other function is the supervisor's role as guide, counsellor and friend. But do midwives still need this statutory prop. Midwifery has progressed considerably since the 1930s. Midwives are now trained to higher education diploma or degree standard. The profession has become more cohesive and it is beginning to assert its identity again.

Of course all professionals need the opportunity to discuss their work and at times seek support for the decisions they have to make. But most people develop these supportive networks around them without the need for a statutory framework. Indeed the more flexible this support is, the more it is likely to meet the real needs of the professional. Isherwood [3] suggests that

'Perhaps we need to elect, or designate, experienced midwives who would be independent of the disciplinary and managerial machinery, with the essential qualities of sympathy and tact, to act as "counsellor and friend".'

An alternative might be to require proper clinical audit conducted among peers where, alongside the continuous monitoring of standards, appropriate professional support will take place underpinned by encouragement and constructive criticism.

## SUMMARY

The supervision of midwives was introduced with the first Midwives Act in 1902 and has remained a statutory requirement ever since.

Changes in midwifery practice and in health service organization since then have led some people to question its current relevance.

The future of supervision may lie in developing a greater role in monitoring standards and, if proved effective, it may be applicable to other professions.

In a service of greater flexibility the process of supervision may need to be streamlined.

## FURTHER ACTION

- Ask your supervisor to talk about her work and how she reconciles the management/supervisory responsibilities she has.

- Arrange a structured discussion among your colleagues using some of the ideas of this chapter. Try to agree the advantages and disadvantages to having supervision. Do not just think about this narrowly in relation to yourselves but consider whether there is a general advantage to the public and the health services.

- See if your discussion group can come to a consensus agreement about whether supervision is a valuable activity in the provision of maternity care.

## REFERENCES

1. Hughes, D. Free Speech: supervisors of midwives. *Midwives Chronicle*. November 1985, **98**, (1174).
2. The *Guardian*, February 3rd 1986.

3. Isherwood, K. Friend or Watchdog? *Nursing Times*, 1988, **84**, (24) June 15th, p. 65.
4. Department of Health. *Working for Patients*. London, HMSO, 1989.
5. Department of Health. *Meeting and Improving Standards in Health Care policy statement on the development of clinical audit*. (Executive Letter EL (93)59), London, DoH, 1993.
6. Landsell, M. Friend and Counsellor. *Nursing Times*, 1989, **85**, (28) July 12th, p. 76.
7. Department of Health. *Assessing the Effects of Health Technologies*. London, DoH, 1992.

# Chapter 4
# The Legal Basis of Health Care

## INTRODUCTION

Almost all maternity care is provided through the National Health Service and consequently most midwives are employed in this sector. The existence of the NHS and the main operating framework of the system are both laid down in legislation dating from the first National Health Service Act 1946 to the most recent Act in 1990. This chapter is designed to increase an understanding of the position of maternity care within this framework, and how midwives may use its structures and processes to improve the provision of maternity care.

## HISTORICAL BACKGROUND

### The new National Health Service

Before 1946 health care in the UK was provided through an unco-ordinated system of hospitals and other services, some publicly maintained by the local authorities, some provided by the charitable and voluntary sector and some by the private sector. It was possible to have free care in the public hospitals but for the most part fees had to be paid for health care. There had been some change to this situation in maternity care with the provision of a paid midwifery service in 1936 and with the statutory obligation upon local authorities to provide a domiciliary maternity service, including payment of the fees of a medical practitioner called in by a midwife.

In 1942, William Beveridge produced a report on the future welfare provision in the UK. It was a report designed to look forward to the end of the Second World War and give promise that the social systems in the country would be improved so that there would be no return to the individual hardships that had been experienced in the years leading up to 1939. One of the commitments of the report was to provide a 'comprehensive national health service which will diminish disease by prevention and cure [1]. The extent to which that was achieved is for the social scientist not the lawyer. But, with great rapidity after the war, the

National Health Service Act was passed in 1946. Figure 4.1 shows the section of the Act relating to midwifery.

The introductory purpose of the Act was

'to provide for the establishment of a comprehensive health service for England and Wales, and for purposes connected therewith'

and the first section outlining the duty of the Minister of Health contained the legal framework for the NHS, the main elements of which were:

- the system would be comprehensive,
- it would be free, and
- its functions would be to improve health and to prevent, diagnose and treat illness.

Section 23 of the Act dealt with the provision of maternity care. For the purposes of the Midwives Acts, each local authority was designated a local health authority and this authority was given the responsibility of ensuring that there would be sufficient midwives in the area it covered to ensure

'attendance on women in their homes as midwives or as maternity nurses during childbirth and from time to time thereafter during a period not less that the lying-in period.'

These local health authorities must not be confused with the authorities we know today. This was simply an administrative re-definition of the existing county or county borough, not a new authority. That was still to come.

The Labour Party at the time published an explanatory leaflet describing the service that would be available under the new arrangements and it said this about the local health authority's responsibility for maternity care:

'They will be responsible for the welfare of expectant and nursing mothers and children under five . . . and their service will include ante- and post-natal clinics, child welfare centres, the supply of supplementary foods (for which they may make charges), and a priority dental service. They will also provide a complete midwifery service for mothers who are confined at home, either by employing midwives themselves or by making arrangements with existing voluntary organisations. Midwives will have the right and the duty to call in doctors in case of need but these doctors must be suitably qualified for maternity work. It will probably not be made one of the duties of the

(4) Regulations may provide, in the case of areas where under PART III.
Part III of the First Schedule to the Education Act, 1944, schemes —*cont.*
of divisional administration relating to the functions of local 7 & 8
education authorities with respect to school health services are in Geo. 6.
force, for the making, variation and revocation of corresponding c. 31.
schemes or divisional administration relating to the functions of
local health authorities under subsection (I) of this section with
respect to the care of children who have not attained the age of five
years and are not attending primary schools maintained by a local
education authority, and the functions of such authorities under
subsection (3) of this section.

(5) A local health authority may, with the approval of the
Minister, contribute to any voluntary organisation formed for any of
the purposes mentioned in subsection (I) of this section.

**23.**—(I) The local health authority shall be the local Midwifery.
supervising authority for the purposes of the Midwives Acts, 1902
to 1936, and accordingly in section eight of the Midwives Acts, 2 Edw. 7.
1902, for the words " council of a county or county borough " c. 17.
there shall be substituted the words " local health authority " and
for the words " said county or county borough " there shall be
substituted the words " said authority ".

(2) It shall be the duty of every local health authority to secure,
whether by making arrangements with Boards of Governors or
teaching hospitals, Hospital Management Committees or voluntary
organisations for the employment by those Boards, Committees or
organisations of certified midwives or by themselves employing
such midwives, that the number of certified midwives so employed
who are available in the authority's area for attendance on women
in their homes as midwives, or as maternity nurses during childbirth
and from time to time thereafter during a period not less than the
lying-in period, is adequate for the needs of the area.

In this subsection the expression " lying-in period " means the
period defined as the lying-in period by any rule for the time being
in force under section three of the Midwives Act, 1902.

(3) Subsection (I) of section nine of the Midwives Act, 1936 26 Geo. 5.
(which enables the Minister to prescribe conditions subject to which &
fees are to be payable by the local health authority to medical I
practitioners called in by midwives) shall have effect as if at the Edw.8.c.40.
end of the subsection there were added the words " including
conditions as to the qualifications of such medical practitioners ".

**Fig. 4.1** Section 23 of the National Health Service Act 1946, showing the
provisions for midwifery.

family doctor to attend his patients in confinement, as most general practitioners are neither interested or sufficiently experienced in obstetrics. But they will be expected to give general medical care to their women patients before and after childbirth. Provision for hospital confinement will no longer be a responsibility of local authorities, but their domiciliary maternity service will include specialist obstetric and gynaecological advice, wherever needed, under arrangements with the Regional Board'. [2]

The Act introduced three separate structures for the provision of health care.

(1) Some services, notably community services, of which midwifery was one along with a home nursing service and a health visiting service, and the ambulance services were to be provided by the county councils acting as local health authorities.

(2) The hospital services were to be administered by Hospital Management Committees or, for teaching hospitals, Boards of Governors. They were to be co-ordinated by Regional Boards.

(3) The general practitioner, dental, optician and pharmacy services continued to practise independently of the NHS but were to offer their services on the basis of a fee-paid contract with a Medical Executive Committee acting on behalf of the NHS.

This tripartite division had considerable implications for maternity care and midwives because it resulted in a lack of continuity of care provisions for the individual woman. If a woman had a homebirth without complications she would receive all her care from the local health authority because she would receive midwife only care. But consider the following situation:

> Susan was pregnant and was to have a homebirth. She had booked for midwife care. She saw her general practitioner for a routine medical examination at the beginning of pregnancy and again at 36 weeks. She also visited her dentist to take advantage of the free dental care she could have during pregnancy. The midwife referred her back to the general practitioner for mild hypertension. He prescribed a mild sedative. The hypertension seemed to settle and the midwife continued to give her care. When labour commenced she was again hypertensive so the midwife arranged for her to go to hospital by ambulance and she delivered at the local hospital. She spent ten days in hospital and was then discharged back to the midwife. Eventually, about six weeks after her delivery, she saw the general practitioner at a postnatal clinic.

In a case such as this, which would not be uncommon, the woman would have received care from all three parts of the health service.

The midwife
The health visitor } Local Health Authority
The ambulance service

The hospital midwife } Hospital Management Committee
The obstetrician

The general practitioner
The pharmacy } Medical Executive Committee
The dentist

Not only was this unsatisfactory for the woman, but it also created boundaries between the different professionals. Any communication between them would not only pass from professional to professional but would need to cross the administrative boundaries of three differently administered systems.

In the unified NHS it is difficult to ensure good communication across different sectors of the same organization. In the original system midwives based in hospital and the community often hardly knew each other's names and rarely, if ever, met.

Although welcomed as the panacea of all ills, it was soon apparent that the original aims of the NHS were unrealistic The great achievement of the NHS then and now was not to produce overnight solutions to illness, but to make available consistent levels of health care service to all people without cost, thus removing for everyone the anxiety of unsupported ill health.

Deficiencies in the system were, however, noted early.

- Costs were not contained, indeed they seemed to rise with increased use of the facilities.
- Standards were not consistent.
- Various hospital enquiries (such as the investigation into the Ely hospital, Cardiff) showed standards of care which were reprehensible, particularly in institutions for the chronically sick and disabled.

However most studies of the new system tended to support its achievements and confirm the *status quo* until 1968 when the Minister of Health published the first in a series of consultation documents spanning the next five years. These identified some of the inherent problems of the current structure. The solution would be found in providing a management structure and ethos and in unifying health care. In 1973 the National Health Service Reorganisation Act was passed and the new structures started operating on 1 April 1974.

## The National Health Service Reorganisation Act 1973

The 1973 Act abolished the existing tripartite system. It transferred the previous responsibilities of the local health authorities to the National Health Service. District midwives, nurses and health visitors changed employer to the NHS. The ambulance services transferred to the responsibility of new Regional Health Authorities. The Medical Executive Committees ceased to exist as separate entities but became committees of the newly formed Area Health Authorities and were renamed the Family Practitioner Committees. There was some debate at the time about the place for social services but these were left with the local authorities.

The structure of the NHS in 1974 is shown in figure 4.2. Hospitals and community services operated at the lowest level of the system, at either health unit or district health authority level. In Scotland the statutory divisions of the structure were known as Health Boards and in Northern Ireland as Health and Social Services Boards.

This Act introduced major change to the midwifery service. All midwives were now employees of the same authority whether in hospital or community and in most places a management structure was introduced that had a head of service over both. It was now possible to manage midwives in an integrated way so that policies and philosophies of care could be adopted throughout the service. At the time it was hoped that systems such as the newly introduced 'domino' schemes might be facilitated by the legislative change. It is now unfortunately clear that the opportunity to introduce a truly flexible system of care by breaking the hospital/community divide within the midwifery service was not grasped at the time.

1974

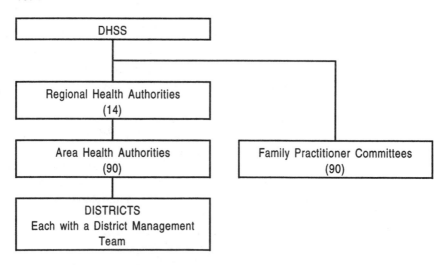

**Fig. 4.2** The structure of the NHS in 1974.

A second change was to make arrangements for the supervision of midwifery to pass to Regional Health Authorities in England, Area Health Authorities in Wales and the Health Boards in Scotland and Northern Ireland.

The 1973 Act also provided an independent voice for the patient in the health care system with the setting up of Community Health Councils. These councils, made up of local councillors and appointees of Regional Health Authorities provided a focus for users of the NHS to raise concerns and complaints about the service.

It became rapidly apparent that the new tiered management structure had too many layers and that decision making was cumbersome. The separation of midwifery practice and the LSA at regional level has been discussed in the previous chapter, but this gulf between the different management levels affected most of the service areas.

## The Health Services Act 1980

Further legislation was introduced in 1980 to streamline the management structure with the abolition of one of the statutory levels (the Area Health Authorities) in England. This new structure was introduced in April 1982.

To manage the service at each level in the organization there was a team of officers who made decisions based upon consensus agreement. In each of these teams was a nurse (or, very occasionally, a midwife in the District Nursing Officer post) who represented the nursing and midwifery interests.

1982

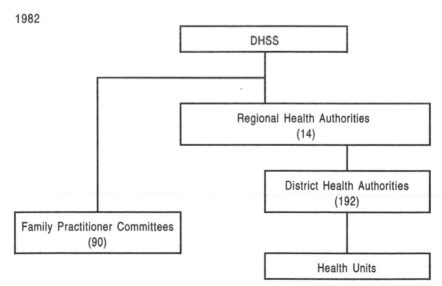

**Fig. 4.3** The structure of the NHS in 1982.

## FUNDING

To understand the magnitude of the changes that were introduced in 1990, it is worth explaining briefly how the funding and management functions were organized between 1980 and 1990.

## Health service funding before 1990

The funding of the health service was very typical of a centrally driven service. The global amount of money that would be available for the health service was, and still is, decided each year in the Government public sector spending round when each spending Ministry negotiates with the Treasury until agreement between all the Ministries is reached about the amount of money available for each. The money for the health service in England was then divided between each of the fourteen Regional Health Authorities on the basis of the services that were available. (Funding arrangements were somewhat different in each of the other countries of the UK which had a global amount for all the services provided and the health 'slice of the cake' was then decided within the country.) The Regional Health Authorities in turn would divide the money to each District Health Authority, again on the basis of the services available. Although there were some mechanisms to weight the money for health and social need, the principle was simple: if a District Health Authority had two hospitals it would receive more money than one that only had one hospital to run. The final part of the financial chain was that the District Health Authority would divide the money out between all the different component service areas for which it was responsible. Each hospital and community service would thus receive appropriate funding. The principle for the hospital was the same as for the District Health Authority. The hospital that had more beds, more functions or more specialities would get more money than one with less.

The Regional Health Authorities were the policy and strategy bodies whilst the District Health Authorities were responsible for the operational management of services. Although management changes such as the introduction of general management and clinical directorates happened afterwards, there was no statutory change suggested until 1989.

## The National Health Service and Community Care Act 1990

During 1987 and 1988 there was a concerted media campaign drawing attention to the lack of funding for the health service. Some professionals were also openly critical of the underfunding. Questions were raised about it in the House of Commons and at Prime Minister's question time. Possibly under this pressure, the Prime Minister, Mrs Thatcher, announced that she would be conducting a Cabinet review of the National Health Service. The report of this review was published as a White Paper, '*Working for Patients*', on 31 January 1989. A fiercely contested Bill passed through Parliament and the Act was passed in 1990. The subsequent NHS changes took place on 1 April 1991.

Before analysing the effect of this Act on the funding of the NHS and maternity services, a brief explanation of the 'community care' part of the Act is worthwhile. A second White Paper had been published in 1989 entitled *Caring for People*. It proposed changes to the provision and funding of care for people with long term health problems (the elderly, the mentally ill and the physically or mentally handicapped) who were being cared for in the community. It involved a changed function for the social services departments of local authorities. The requirements of the two White Papers were combined into the 1990 Act, the second part of which, despite its title, has little relevance to maternity care.

There was however something of relevance to midwifery in *Working for Patients*. As well as indicating the statutory changes that the Government intended, the White Paper also described some of the policy directions that the Government wished to see, even though they would not be formalized in law. An example of this was the intention to require medical audit. There was little mention of the health care professionals other than doctors in the White Paper, but notably it drew attention to midwives.

> 'As part of this initiative, local managers, in consultation with their professional colleagues, will be expected to re-examine all areas of work to identify the most cost effective use of professional skills. This may involve a reappraisal of traditional patterns and practices. Examples include the extended role of nurses to cover specific duties normally undertaken by junior doctors ... and making full use of midwives as recommended in the reports of the Maternity Services Advisory Committee.' [3]

The introduction to the Act states its purpose to:

> 'make further provision about health authorities and Family Practitioner Committees; to provide for the establishment of National Health Service trusts; to make further provision about the financing of the practices of medical practitioners; to amend Part III of the Local Government Finance Act 1982; to amend the National Health Service Act 1977 and the National Health Service (Scotland) Act 1984; to make further provision concerning the provision of accommodation and other welfare services by local authorities and the powers of the Secretary of State as respects the social services functions of such authorities; to repeal the Health Services Act 1976; and for connected purposes.'

Ideologically the change introduced by the 1990 Act was almost as revolutionary as the original 1946 Act which created the National Health Service. Prior to 1991, the NHS was a centrally organized service which in many ways mirrored the workings of the command economies of the communist states of Central and Eastern Europe before their recent changes. That in itself was surprising in that it existed in a predominantly free market economy regardless of the political complexion of the Government of the day.

The 1990 Act introduced into the health care system an element of the market economy by creating an 'internal market'.

## An explanation of the NHS internal market

A free market economy is one in which the economic functions of trade – buying and selling – and the distribution of economic resources, for example labour and capital, are not controlled, but operate independently. An example of this would be the operation of the high street retail shop. No-one tells the company what goods to stock and no-one directs customers to one shop rather than another. People choose to shop where they want and buy what they want. The shop keeper stocks what he thinks they want. He can do this by monitoring what they buy; but, more importantly, he can try to make his shop more attractive to customers than those of his competitors and he can try to influence their buying habits by advertising. Compare this with the old Soviet command economy where the Moscow state shop, GUM, stocked what the government told it to at set prices and people had no choice but to shop there.

Until 1991 the health service was paradoxically run on command economy lines whilst the general economic framework in the UK was a free market.

A free market health care system is one where there is no nationally provided system and people are free to find their own health care from whichever providers they choose, and they pay for this care when needed or by taking out insurance. Like goods in a shop, care is available if the person has the money, but if not then he does not have access to it. The prime example of this is the current system in the United States where most people enjoy a very high standard of health care supported by private insurance but 37 million people are denied access to it because they are too poor.

This short digression into economic theory has been necessary to understand what the 1990 Act introduced.

The Act did not abolish the National Health Service. It still retains the important first requirement of the Secretary of State, and therefore the government, to provide a comprehensive health care system. It does not require people to fund their health care directly but continues to fund it by raising general taxation. The original principle of providing care equitably and free at the point of need is retained. What the Act does is to introduce elements of the free market economy within the system itself.

Remember the previous description of the financing mechanisms for the health service, with money passing down the chain of command to hospital level dependent upon the services that each level provided. Now, money is apportioned to the Regional Health Authorities and District Health Authorities on the basis of the population they cover. It is divided out taking account of population numbers with some additional assessment made to take account of each population's health status and therefore health needs. At District Health Authority level there is now a very different mechanism for funding the hospitals and other direct service providers. The care is now purchased and there is no automatic transfer of money without an agreement about the level of service that will be provided.

## Buying health care

The new Act created within the health service, 'buyers' of health care.

### The District Health Authority

The District Health Authority's principal responsibilities are to assess the health care needs of the population it serves and to purchase the appropriate care to meet these needs. The statutory officers of the District Health Authority are:

- a chairman appointed by the Secretary of State,
- five executive members which must include the chief officer of the Authority, and
- five non-executive members, who are not employed by the NHS but are appointed.

There have already been changes to these authorities. A number of them have amalgamated and are now commonly calling themselves commissioning agencies rather than health authorities.

### The fund holding general practice

This was a completely new funding mechanism introduced by the Act. Group practices with over 7000 on their lists (it was originally 11 000 but this requirement was reduced) could apply to receive money directly from a regional allocation to buy health care for the people on their list. It was not mandatory. Practices could apply for fund holding status and were assessed for suitability.

The services that these practices could purchase were restricted to:

- out-patient services, including diagnostic and treatment costs;
- a defined group of in-patient and day case treatments such as hip replacements and cataract removals, for which there may be some choice over the time and place of treatment; and
- diagnostic tests, such as X-ray examination and pathology tests, which are undertaken by hospitals at the direct request of general practitioners.

Since the Act was passed the services that general practitioner fundholders may purchase have been extended by regulation to include community nursing and health visiting services. The general practitioner fundholder still may not purchase maternity services or midwifery services on behalf of his patients.

### Selling health care

On the other side of the internal market are providers of health care. These are all the institutions, units and services actually providing direct care, the hospitals, community services and ambulance services.

On the passing of the 1990 Act all these services were still directly managed by the District Health Authorities. The Act introduced the mechanism for breaking this managerial link between what were to be two sides of a purchasing arrangement – the buyer and the seller. This was the new NHS Trust. Services or institutions could apply for Trust status and if this was agreed would be entrusted with running their own affairs whilst still remaining within the NHS. They would be managed by a Board of Directors, with a chairman, executive and non-executive members. The executive members would include the chief executive, a medical director, the senior nurse manager and a finance director. Current NHS Trusts are each made up of 11 members including the chairman who is appointed by the Secretary of State.

To become a Trust, a hospital or other service must produce a prospectus in support of its application and submit this to the Regional Health Authority. The Regional Health Authority must conduct a public consultation and advise the Secretary of State on whether to accept the application. The Secretary of State gives final approval.

An NHS Trust independently manages its own affairs. The White Paper proposed:

'to give NHS Hospital Trusts a range of powers and freedoms which are not, and will not be, available to health authorities generally. Greater freedom will stimulate greater enterprise and commitment, which will in turn improve services for patients. NHS Hospital Trusts will be a novel part of a system of hospital care alongside health authority-managed and private sector hospitals, and will increase the range of choice available to patients and their GPs.' [3]

Another important freedom was the opportunity to 'settle the pay and conditions of their staff, including doctors, nurses and others covered by national pay review bodies.' They would be able to decide whether to follow national pay agreements or not. The Act safeguarded staff who were employees when a new Trust was set up by protecting their original pay and conditions. The staff's right to belong the NHS superannuation scheme was also safeguarded.

It was also made clear that care for health service patients could, if financially competitive, be purchased from the private sector.

In summary, the Act introduced

| Purchasers | Providers |
|---|---|
| District Health Authorities | DHA managed units |
| General practitioner fund holders | NHS Trusts |
| | The private sector |

The element of competition that always exists when people can buy and sell what and how they please is encouraged by this new configuration of the services as neither District Health Authorities nor general practitioner fund holders are restricted in their choice of health care provider, whether those providers are within or outside their geographical area. The purchasing of health care has no boundaries and care can be provided from whichever source provides the appropriate level of care for the most acceptable price. Not unlike the high street market, except NHS purchasers are obtaining health care on behalf of the users of the service rather than the users obtaining it directly for themselves.

## The NHS contract

There is a third element in any buying and selling activity, the contract that exists between the parties.

It is open for any purchasing authority or provider unit to enter a normal contract with a third party to provide services. These contracts are enforceable in law and it is open to either party who believes that there has been a breach in the contract to go to court to enforce the contract or seek damages. Any contract between an independent midwife or practice and the health service would fall into this category. The first such contract was agreed in 1994 between the South East London Midwifery Group Practice and its local purchasing authorities as a pilot scheme.

However the 1990 Act introduced a special form of contract, the 'NHS contract'. This is described in section 4 of the Act as an 'arrangement under which one health service body ... arranges for the provision to it by another health service body ... of goods or services which it reasonably requires for the purposes of its functions'.

In non-statutory language, an NHS contract is the agreement made between a purchaser and a provider. These contracts are not enforceable in law but when there is a dispute over the terms of an agreement Regional Health Authorities and ultimately the Secretary of State for Health will be called upon to adjudicate.

The Act listed those 'bodies' which can be party to an NHS contract. These are:

- a health authority;
- a health board;
- the Common Services Agency for the Scottish Health Authority;
- a Family Practitioner Services Authority;
- an NHS Trust;
- a recognized fund holding practice;
- the Dental Practice Board or the Scottish Dental Practice Board;
- the Public Health Laboratory Service Board; and
- the Secretary of State.

Figure 4.4 illustrates the current structure of the NHS.

The application of the new system varies in different localities but to give a general idea of how it works in principle it is described in the following case study.

### Case study: maternity care in Rosebank Health Authority

Rosebank Health Authority has given its Department of Public Health the responsibility for purchasing health care for the needs of its population, including maternity care. Figure 4.5 shows the health authority and the maternity services accessible to it.

The department first analyses the needs of women for maternity care for the next year. To do this, it has access to routine data from previous birth notifications, from hospital data and from the Office of Population, Census and Surveys which publishes birth-related information including birth trends. From this information it estimates the anticipated number of deliveries including anticipated complications.

From this analysis, Rosebank estimates that there will be 4000 deliveries in the population it serves and that there will be a 12% caesarean section rate, an 8% forceps rate, 5% of babies will need special care and 1% will require neonatal intensive care at a regionally based unit.

The department then decides the standard of care it would like to purchase on behalf of the population. To do this it it asks one of the researchers in the department, who is a midwife specializing in audit, to

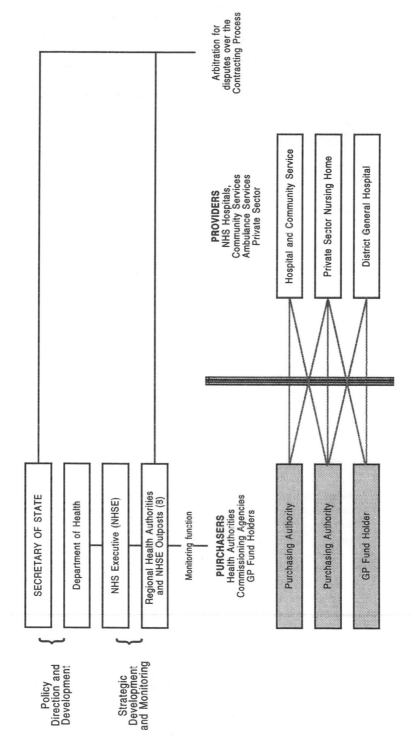

**Fig. 4.4** The structure of the NHS in 1992.

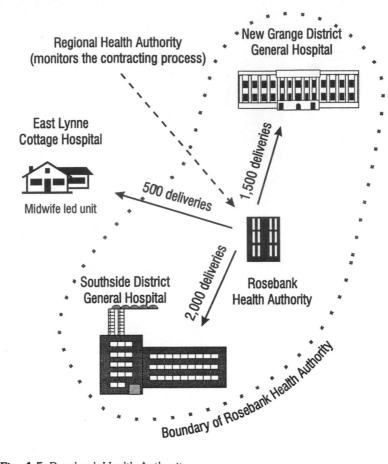

**Fig. 4.5** Rosebank Health Authority.

research and report on the optimal standard of care that should be provided. It also consults with senior obstetricians, midwives and general practitioners working in the local provider units to build up a picture of current good practice and what can reasonably be expected from any maternity service. It knows that it must demand the best possible care in any contract with provider units, but it must at the same time not demand a standard that is impossible to achieve. The balance can be difficult.

Finally, the purchaser will try to find out from the users of the service what sort of service they would like to receive, including where they would like to deliver. Analysis of past patient satisfaction surveys and examination of general practitioner referral patterns will give the department an idea of this.

When all this information is put together, the Rosebank Authority issues a service specification outlining the amount and standard of maternity care it would like to purchase. Figure 4.6 shows the table of contents from a typical service specification.

---

# MATERNITY SERVICES

## SERVICE SPECIFICATION

## TABLE OF CONTENTS

---

**Fig. 4.6** Part of a typical service specification for maternity services.

Meanwhile, Southside and Newgrange hospital maternity services and the midwife led unit at East Lynne have prepared business plans which set out their intended services. It is clear that the three services can meet the needs of the Rosebank Authority and after a period of negotiation over the money that the authority will pay and the standard it wishes to purchase, it formally agrees to purchase 2000 deliveries from Southside, 1500 from Newgrange and 500 from East Lynne. During the year it then monitors the effectiveness of the contracts it has entered into.

This is a very simplistic model of the NHS contracting system but shows clearly the importance of having some influence over the development of service specifications, business plans and the monitoring of the subsequent NHS contracts. All these activities affect the way midwives are expected to offer their services. They should ensure that they have an input into these vital stages.

## MATERNITY CARE AND THE NEW NHS ARRANGEMENTS

As with every other service, the maternity services will be subjected to the NHS contracting process and purchasing authorities will be required to find out what maternity care is needed by the population. They are also increasingly requiring care to be effective and incorporating these principles into their service requirements, and at the same time demanding that ineffective care should be discontinued. This is likely to become a powerful mechanism for change and this potential is demonstrated in the recent policy documents on maternity care.

The 1993 Government consultation document, *Changing Childbirth* [4] proposed radical change in the provision of maternity care. It suggested that purchasing authorities should build requirements for change into their service specifications. Following the consultation a letter was circulated by the NHS Executive asking purchasers to

'draw up plans for *Changing Childbirth*, and ensure that its recommendations are reflected in both their 3–5 year purchasing strategies and their 1995/96 purchasing plans ... This will help to develop a staged programme for the implementation team and enable outliers to be monitored closely, having regard to the degree of change required and the resources available.'

There should however be a word of caution about the extent to which the new system has improved choices for women. There is some evidence that women's opportunities to choose the hospital where they want to have their babies are being limited by the narrow interpretation of agreed contracting arrangements, so that they may only go to a hospital with which their local purchasing authority has a contract.

The importance of midwives becoming involved in the purchasing activity, and particularly the development of purchasing strategies and service specifications, cannot be stressed enough. Their advice will be invaluable to managers in both the purchasing and providing sectors of the health service and they should see this as an opportunity to develop their practice and the service they give to women. They should also be aware of any difficulty experienced by a client in choosing where to have her baby and should make this known, through their managers, to the purchasing authority.

## SUMMARY

The structure of the National Health Service and the provision of health care is controlled by statute.

There have been a number of major re-organizations of care over the past 20 years but the most recent, a result of the National Health Service and Community Care Act 1990, has been the most radical.

Opportunities exist within the new system of health care purchasing both for midwives to develop their practice and for more responsive care to be given to women.

## FURTHER ACTION

- Ask for a copy of the last service specification for maternity care.

- Discuss with your managers how to make the midwifery contribution to purchasing strategies and service specifications effective.

- With colleagues discuss the proposals in *Changing Childbirth* and draw up your own strategy for their implementation within the required timetable.

## REFERENCES

1. Beveridge, W. *Social Insurance and Allied Services. The Beveridge Report.* London, HMSO, 1942.
2. Fitzgerald, H. *A Guide to the NHS Act 1946.* London, The Labour Party, 1946/7.
3. Department of Health. *Working for Patients.* London, HMSO, 1989.
4. Department of Health. *Changing Childbirth: the Report of the Expert Maternity Group (Executive Letter EL (93)72),* London, DoH 1994.

# Chapter 5
# When Things go Wrong

All practising midwives know that things can go wrong sometimes: the pregnancy that becomes complicated, the unexpected stillbirth, the postnatal infection. In most of these situations the staff looking after the woman are clearly not at fault. There may however be times when they appear to have contributed to the problem. Sometimes the problem is not clinical but may be a complaint about their manner or their failure to communicate. In these circumstances patients have the right to seek redress and they may turn to two possible legal processes.

If they believe the professional has been guilty of misconduct they may report this to the relevant statutory body; if they believe that the professional has been negligent they may turn to the legal system for help.

Any midwife involved in either of these processes will find it difficult. She may be the person 'accused' of a professional misdemeanour or she may be called as a witness in either a professional conduct hearing or a legal case. No book on the law can take away the feeling of distress and anxiety when these things happen particularly when they may be connected with a distressing outcome of a pregnancy. However, knowing how the systems work and where to get help and support can be invaluable.

Each system has its own characteristics and the outcome for the midwife can be very different, but there are certain things that both the statutory body processes and the legal processes have in common. First, both can take a long time and, secondly, they are designed to be fair to both parties. Whether fairness is achieved or not is sometimes challenged but the complicated way in which cases are prepared and then heard has been developed over time so that all sides of a case can be fully explored.

## PROFESSIONAL CONDUCT

Chapter 2 described the statutory requirements for the regulation of the professional conduct of the nurse, midwife and health visitor. The two-tier system of professional screening prior to referral to the Professional

Conduct Committee is designed to protect the midwife from untoward allegations. The hearing itself follows legal procedure thus allowing a full examination of the case from both sides. The midwife through her representative will have the opportunity to explain her position fully to the Committee. The whole process is nevertheless daunting and complicated. The following hypothetical case gives both the facts of a case as well as the varying interpretations that can be drawn from the facts. It shows just how difficult it can be for the Professional Conduct Committee when trying to decide whether a midwife is guilty of professional misconduct or not.

### Case Study: the unexpected delivery

#### The facts

Mary was admitted to her local hospital in labour. Jenny, a midwife, examined her, told her she was in early labour and that she, Jenny, would be looking after her during the night. Jenny took observations about every half an hour but did not stay in the room with Mary. The labour progressed very quickly and at one stage Mary called for Jenny saying she thought she would be having the baby soon. Jenny examined her and said she thought it would be some time. She left the room. About 15 minutes later Mary delivered without a midwife and with only her husband to help.

#### Mary's version

I went to the hospital when I was having contractions every five minutes. The midwife who saw me first seemed to be preoccupied and, although she examined me well, was in a hurry to get away. She did come in and out of my room to listen to my baby's heartbeat and check on me but, when suddenly my labour seemed to get out of control, I had to call her to see me. She examined me and told me I wasn't going to have my baby for some time. I told her I thought she was wrong and my husband and I asked her to stay. We both thought I was going to have the baby very soon. I was very frightened when she left. Suddenly I had a very strong urge to push and within seconds my baby was born. We rang the call bell but no-one came until it was all over. My baby is fine but the whole experience was dreadful and I don't think the midwife took any of my concerns seriously. It is her job to help me have my baby and what should have been a lovely experience turned out to be a nightmare.

#### Jenny's version

I came onto night duty and the labour ward was very full. I was asked to look after a woman who had had a previous caesarean section. There was only one other midwife on duty as one midwife who should have been on that night had rung in to say she was sick. Mary was admitted in labour and I was assigned to look after her as well as the other woman. I admitted her and everything seemed to be straightforward. She was having her second baby; her husband was with her. She seemed to be coping well with the contractions and all her recordings were fine. I went in about every half an hour to check on her. I should have gone in more often but the other case was very difficult and she was needing a lot of support. Mary rang and said that she thought she was going to have her baby very soon. I examined her and the cervix was 5cm dilated. I didn't think she would deliver quickly. My mind was on the other woman who was bleeding slightly and I needed to discuss this urgently with the registrar. I reassured Mary and left. About 15 minutes later I heard her ringing her bell and went to her. She had just delivered. I was very surprised. I certainly did not expect it. Had I done so I would have stayed with her and passed the other problem to the midwife who was on with me.

### The Outcome

Mary felt so unhappy about her treatment she complained to the hospital and also wrote to the UKCC complaining personally about Jenny's professional conduct. Jenny was notified by letter that the UKCC had received a complaint about her. In her case the facts had been looked at by the Preliminary Proceedings Committee which had decided to close the case with a caution as to future conduct. This meant that there would be no further action. If the Preliminary Proceedings Committee had decided to refer the case, it would have raised some difficult questions of professional accountability.

The stories are very different. Mary feels cheated of a happy delivery; Jenny feels she did everything she could have given the circumstances. Had it gone to the Professional Conduct Committee, the Committee would have had to consider a number of questions:

- Should Jenny have done something about the situation she was in by referring it to the manager so that Mary would have the care she was entitled to?

- Should she have been more alert to Mary's assessment of her labour even when the examination seemed to contradict it?

- Does her failure to give optimum care in the circumstances amount to professional misconduct?

In order to ensure that her case is fairly considered, given the complexity of the possible interpretations, Jenny would be well advised to seek professional support as soon as she knows that there is an allegation of misconduct against her.

## What to do when misconduct is alleged

The first and understandable feelings of any midwife who has been reported to the UKCC for alleged professional misconduct or because her health may be affecting her standards of practice are likely to be disbelief, followed by a sense of panic. If the local supervising authority has suspended her, it has a duty under the Midwives Rules to notify her of the decision to suspend and the reason. However, if an individual, a client, a fellow midwife or other professional colleague, has reported an alleged offence to the UKCC, the midwife may have no such notification. It will be considered by the Preliminary Proceedings Committee and only when that Committee has made a decision will the midwife hear of the complaint. In some instances the Preliminary Proceedings Committee will have found there is no case to answer and the midwife will simply be told this, without any further details. For some midwives this is a satisfactory process as they only hear about the complaint when it has been dismissed, thus saving weeks of worry before it is considered by the Preliminary Proceedings Committee. For others the knowledge that a complaint against them has been considered without their knowledge is unacceptable.

## Complaints through the LSA

Most of the serious complaints come through the local supervising authority, and are likely to be preceded by an investigation by a supervisor of midwives. The supervisor may ask for a written statement from the midwife as part of the investigation and may also ask for statements from anyone else who may have been involved. The LSA may suspend the midwife on the basis of the investigation, and may require the midwife to attend an interview with the 'representative' of the LSA. This person may not always be a midwife, but a regional nurse. If accepted good practice is followed (and there is no statutory requirement to do so) this nurse will be fully advised by a supervisor of midwives and will facilitate a detailed and fair discussion with the midwife concerned.

There is no right to representation at such an interview as there is in a disciplinary hearing, but the midwife is strongly advised to contact her professional organization or trade union before submitting any personal statement in writing and before going to any interview. She should be accompanied and, if the LSA questions this, she should ask her organization to organize it for her. **This is usually not the time to act alone**. Anger and worry can impair the judgment of even the most rational of people. As it is her professional practice which is in question, assistance at these interviews is often best provided by another midwife from the professional organization.

If on investigation the LSA decides to suspend the midwife and report her to the UKCC, it must notify her of this decision in writing giving the reasons for doing so.

### Consideration by the Preliminary Proceedings Committee

The case will then be considered by the Preliminary Proceedings Committee. This is a difficult time. The Preliminary Proceedings Committee does not see the midwife, unless it is considering a complaint about her health. It may write asking for a response to the allegations made, which will be summarized in the letter.

There are three 'rules' here.

- First, co-operate. It is not in the best interests of the midwife to obstruct the investigation.
- Second, keep in constant touch with the professional organization and do nothing without its advice.
- Third, do not try to influence the other people who are involved in the investigation.

The midwife is likely to be advised to keep away from her place of work, and this she should do. She and her representative are very likely to need documentary evidence to help with the case – clinical records, staffing levels, corroborative evidence from others – but this should be arranged by the representative rather than the midwife.

If the Preliminary Proceedings Committee decides that there is an allegation which should be considered by the Professional Conduct Committee, the midwife will be informed in writing at this stage with a Notice of Proceedings which also sets out the intended charges. A formal response to these charges should be made, again with professional help, as it is still possible at this stage for the Preliminary Proceedings Committee to decide not to proceed.

### Before the Professional Conduct Committee

If a hearing is to take place, the midwife has a right to representation and is strongly advised to have this. The hearing can take place in the absence of the midwife but, however much attending a hearing causes anxiety, the midwife is also strongly advised to be there. Even if she is found guilty of misconduct, she will have the opportunity to speak in mitigation. There are a number of cases where the Professional Conduct Committee takes no action even when misconduct is proved. Examples of this are given in a UKCC booklet, *Complaints about Professional Conduct*, and include cases where:

- the incident was isolated and uncharacteristic and the practitioner appears to have learnt lessons from it, or
- there were, at the time, overwhelming personal problems which led

the practitioner to behave inappropriately and which have been resolved. [1]

It is possible for a representative to explain matters such as these, but it is much better for the midwife to do it herself.

# What to do on removal from the Register

The midwife removed from part 10 of the Register may not practise as a midwife. She may be on other parts of the Register from which she has not been removed and in these circumstances may continue to practise using her alternative qualifications. However, her name may be removed from all parts of the Register and she will have effectively lost her livelihood.

### Immediate help

She may receive practical, immediate advice from her professional organization. In the first instance this may be guidance on whether to appeal against the decision. There is a right of appeal to the High Court although this right is not automatic. The professional organization should advise whether an appeal is possible or likely to succeed.

Once removed from the Register the midwife may be ineligible for continuing membership of her professional organization. There is a voluntary organization, which is partially supported in its activities by the main professional organizations and which is able to offer support, counselling and advice in these circumstances – the Nurses Welfare Society.

### Restoration to the Register

In the long term, the midwife may wish to have her name restored to the Register. This is almost a 'Catch 22' situation. To restore a name the UKCC prefers to have evidence that the practitioner is 'rehabilitated'. If her name has been removed on health grounds, then favourable medical reports should suffice. If the grounds were based on the standard of practice, it is not possible to show that practice is improved as she is no longer in practice.

It may be advisable to choose to do some form of job or activity which could be used as a proxy for midwifery practice. Obtaining work as a health care assistant, doing voluntary care or becoming active in a maternity related organization such as the National Childbirth Trust would all be considered favourably. Particularly work with the National Childbirth Trust, as it applies rigorous standards to its volunteers and the training it gives could be invaluable.

The real point of this is that the UKCC does not like removing names from the Register and usually wishes to restore them as soon as possible but it must have some indication that the midwife will in future offer a safe standard of care. Although it is not particularly useful to compare the general requirements relating to nurses and midwives, the fact that a midwife may practise completely independently of the controls usually inherent in being employed must make the UKCC cautious about restoration without evidence of improvement.

## LITIGATION

The case of Mary and Jenny described earlier ended without mishap. Both Mary and her baby were healthy even if Mary was unhappy with the management of her labour. But what might have happened if the baby had been born, needed resuscitation and was subsequently found to be brain damaged?

This section will use the same case but this time Mary's baby had birth asphyxia and was brain damaged. Mary would be faced with many years looking after a handicapped child. The child may need considerable resources to help him with even basic functions. Their home may need adaptations and she and her husband may need to pay for extra help. This situation could last for many years and without extra resources it would be very difficult for the whole family. For all these reasons she is likely to consider a civil action claiming that Jenny was negligent.

### What is negligence?

Negligence is either an action or a failure to act which breaches a duty of care held towards someone and which results in damage. In a famous judgment (*Donoghue* v. *Stevenson* (1932)), Lord Atkin said

> 'You must take reasonable care to avoid acts or omissions which you can reasonably foresee would be likely to injure your neighbour. Who, then, in law is my neighbour? The answer seems to be – persons who are so closely and directly affected by my act that I ought reasonably to have them in contemplation as being so affected when I am directing my mind to the acts or omissions which are called in question.'

For a negligence case to be successful three things have to be proved:

- that the defendant had a duty of care towards her client;
- that the duty of care was breached; and
- that the breach of the duty of care caused the damage.

# The duty of care

In the case of Mary and Jenny, Mary would have no difficulty in proving that Jenny had a duty of care towards her. Anyone who offers themselves as skilled in medicine, midwifery, nursing or any other paramedical activity has an accepted duty that arises independently of any contractual arrangements there may also be. A patient or client of a health care professional will be defined by the courts as the 'neighbour' described in Lord Atkin's judgment.

This is not the case if someone requires medical or midwifery help in an emergency and where there is no pre-existing relationship between the person and the professional.

At one level, this is easy to understand. If a midwife is out shopping and sees a woman about to deliver her baby there is no obligation in law for her to go and help. There is no duty of care between them. However, if the woman was one of her clients, she would have a duty towards her.

The situation is more complicated for the midwife working in the community. Again she has a duty towards her clients and this would extend to emergency treatment for them, if requested, even if she were off duty. But what if the midwife is called out to see a woman in an emergency who lives in the area but has not booked for maternity services? In this circumstance, the fact that the midwife is employed to give maternity care and that there is a statutory obligation upon the health service to provide that care (discussed more fully in Chapter 8) means that there is a pre-existing relationship, even if indirect, and the midwife will have a legal duty of care.

The other test for the existence of a duty of care is whether the professional has been asked to give assistance. It is probable that if a man had a heart attack outside a general practitioner's surgery the doctor would not be obliged to help, but if someone came into the surgery and asked for the help of a doctor he would then have a duty of care to act in the emergency and failure to do so would be a breach of that duty.

# The breach of the duty of care

Returning to the case of Mary and Jenny, it is likely there would be consensus that Jenny breached her duty of care to Mary. Mary delivered alone even though she had alerted a member of staff that she thought she was going to have her baby.

To achieve a consensus about whether a professional has failed to give proper care requires an assessment of what the expected standard of care should be in the first place, so that it can then be judged whether someone has fallen below that standard. The law has developed a set of rules on the expected standard of care which enable consistent decisions to be made.

## The expected standard of care

When describing negligence, Lord Atkin said that reasonable care should be exercised towards one's neighbour. Reasonably the professional is expected to offer a standard of care above that of the ordinary man. But what should that level be?

The legal test to decide on the required standard was defined in the case of *Bolam* v. *Friern Hospital Management Committee* (1957).

> Mr Bolam was admitted to hospital to have electro-convulsive therapy. During the treatment he suffered fractures and subsequently claimed that these could have been avoided if he had had relaxant drugs and had been restrained properly. He also said that he should have been told of the risk of fractures. The expert witnesses agreed that there was a large body of competent doctors who would not use relaxants for the procedure.

In the judgment it was said:

> 'where you get a situation which involves the use of some special skill or competence, then the test as to whether there has been negligence or not is not the test of the man on the top of a Clapham omnibus, because he has not got this special skill. The test is the standard of the ordinary skilled man exercising and professing to have that special skill . . . It is a well established law that it is sufficient if he exercises the ordinary skill of an ordinary competent man exercising that particular art . . . A doctor is not guilty of negligence if he has acted in accordance with a practice accepted as proper by a responsible body of medical men skilled in that particular art.'

This case is important in that these are the rules on which the courts decide what is a reasonable standard of care. It happened to be a case involving doctors but applies equally to all other professional staff, including midwives.

It also highlights the important role of the expert witness in any negligence case. More and more, as the courts accept the multi-professional involvement in these cases, the skill of a midwife may be questioned and the expert witnesses will be midwives. The court does not expect these midwives to be drawn from the best practitioners, but rather that they should present what a responsible body of ordinary practitioners would do given the circumstances of the case.

Even though the rules laid down in the *Bolam* case are fairly definitive, this does not mean that the outcome of a case is always predictable. Both sides in the trial will have expert witnesses and the judges often have to draw a conclusion by balancing the two sets of opinions.

Another problem that arises when trying to decide what the expected professional standard should be is that cases are often decided many years after the clinical events have taken place. The rule is also followed that the standard of clinical care should be that which prevailed at the time of the events, even if it would no longer be acceptable at the time of the trial.

Take another case, that of *Whitehouse v. Jordon and Another* (1981).

> Mrs Whitehouse was a small woman but in pregnancy it was decided that she should have a trial of labour. In January 1970 she was admitted to hospital in labour. Mr Jordon, the senior registrar, decided on a trial of forceps to see whether she could deliver vaginally. After pulling for five or six contractions he decided to do a caesarean section. The baby was born apnoeic and required prolonged resuscitation. He (Stuart) was subsequently brain damaged and, acting through his mother, sued Mr Jordon claiming that he had pulled too hard and for too long on the forceps.

The opinion of the judge at the trial was that Mr Jordon was negligent. The Court of Appeal reversed the decision and it passed to the House of Lords where the case was eventually dismissed by a majority vote of the Law Lords of three to two. The final judgment was not reached until 1981 when Stuart was eleven years old. The decision was made on an assessment of whether a body of responsible doctors would have done what Mr Jordon did, but it had to refer back to 1970 when trial of forceps was used much more commonly than in 1981 when it had largely been abandoned. The way in which the case progressed through all the court levels and was eventually decided only on a majority vote indicates the fine balance of the final decision.

Another important case which has further clarified the standard of care expected also arose in the maternity services. In *Wilsher v. Essex Area Health Authority* (1988) the principle was accepted that a doctor's duty of care can be assessed in relation to the post he holds. Again this would apply equally to midwives.

> Baby Martin Wilsher was born prematurely. He had respiratory difficulties and required oxygen. A senior house officer wrongly inserted a catheter into the umbilical vein instead of the artery. He arranged for an X-ray to check its position and asked the registrar if he would also check its position. Neither doctor saw that it was wrongly sited for over 24 hours. Subsequently Martin suffered retrolental fibroplasia and is partially sighted.

The Health Authority was found to be negligent but in the judge's summing up he added that, whilst the registrar was negligent, the senior house officer was not. He was entitled to rely on having his work checked as he was in a learning post.

This is important for three reasons which also apply to midwives.

(1) When a midwife is in a learning position, perhaps learning a new skill, she is entitled to have her practice supervised.

(2) The student midwife also has the right to proper supervision and it will be the midwife, like the registrar, who could be found negligent if she does not exercise proper supervision over the student.

(3) The employer is bound to provide sufficient supervision for trainees and, if it does not, it can be found independently negligent.

## Did the breach of the duty of care cause the damage?

Finally, in the case of Mary and Jenny, did Jenny's failure to give care cause the damage to Mary's baby? It may be very much more difficult for Mary's lawyers to prove this final vital link, that Mary's baby was left handicapped because she delivered without professional support. Were there antenatal reasons why the baby was handicapped? Had the baby been deprived of oxygen in early labour before Mary had come into hospital? Would the baby have been born damaged even if Jenny had been with Mary throughout the labour?

The difficulty in proving this causal link is very clear in the case of *Barnett v. Chelsea and Kensington Hospital Management Committee* (1969).

> Three night watchmen went to a hospital casualty department at about eight o'clock in the morning. They had been vomiting and one, Mr Barnett, was ill enough to need to lie down. The nurse contacted the casualty officer who was himself ill and told him about the three men. He suggested that they go home and if necessary see their own doctors. Later that day Mr Barnett died. It was found that he and the others had arsenical poisoning. Mrs Barnett sued for damages.

The court found that the casualty officer had a duty of care towards Mr Barnett and that in failing to see him and admit him to the hospital, he had breached that duty.

Nevertheless Mrs Barnett lost the case because the judges failed to accept a link between the failures of the doctor and the Hospital Management Committee and Mr Barnett's death. Arsenic poisoning is very rare and it would have been impossible to obtain the antidote even if an accurate diagnosis had been made. Mr Barnett's death was therefore ascribed to the poisoning rather than to the negligence.

### Causation in midwifery and obstetric practice

There are times when the link between the damage someone has suffered and a negligent act is very apparent, and this applies in midwifery and obstetrics as in any other specialty. A pack left inside the vagina causing infection, a swab left in the abdomen at operation or a baby injured at delivery by a scalpel or episiotomy scissors are so clearly things that should not have happened that the court will readily recognize the causal link. In all other cases it is for the plaintiff to prove the link, on the balance of probabilities, between the negligent action or omission and the damage that occurred.

There are particular circumstances in obstetrics that make it more difficult to define this causal link. Many of the cases are ones in which the fetus has sustained the alleged damage rather than the mother. Much of the care and monitoring of the fetus remains indirect. Courts are, therefore, often required to make a judgment about whether a fetus has been damaged by a very particular act, omission or set of circumstances based only upon indirect observations, or by looking backwards from the time of delivery (or even some time afterwards) and assuming that a child's condition was caused by those circumstances.

### Events in labour – particular clinical issues associated with causation

The courts currently place emphasis on the examination of labour records and cardiotocograph (CTG) tracings when trying to decide whether there has been negligence on the part of the midwife. Indeed one of the most common reasons for a case to be brought is failure to monitor the condition of the fetus in labour.

Some doubts have, however, been raised about the link between events occurring in labour and subsequent brain damage. In the Royal College of Midwives' William Power Memorial lecture in November 1991 [2] the then Chief Medical Officer, Sir Donald Acheson, discussed the possibility that much subsequently diagnosed brain damage could be the result of events taking place antenatally rather than in labour. This idea is gaining strength among doctors and midwives but has not as yet influenced court decisions on negligence. Whether recognition of the influence of antenatal rather than intranatal management will result in less litigation is still not known, but it may, of course, just shift the legal emphasis to questioning care in pregnancy rather than care in labour.

The courts are influenced by varying interpretations of the CTG when making a judgment. However, there is growing clinical controversy over the interpretation of these graphs, particularly if the monitoring is not accompanied by fetal blood analysis. The extent to which CTG abnormalities can be linked to fetal compromise is now much less certain. This is a continuing clinical debate and when a CTG recording is available for examination by the courts, its characteristics still play an important part in the adjudication process.

## Vicarious liability

In most of the cases given so far, the defendants have been health authorities rather than a named professional. This is possible because of the doctrine of vicarious liability by which the law can hold one person or institution liable for the actions of another. The most common form of vicarious liability is that of an employer held responsible for the negligent actions of employees in the course of their employment.

The National Health Service accepts vicarious liability thus indemnifying its employees for their negligent actions. This has been the situation since the first days of the NHS for midwives and nurses, although it was not until the early 1990s that this liability was extended to doctors employed by the NHS. The general practitioner, contracted to the NHS, remains personally liable for any claims made against him.

NHS Trusts are required in the 1990 legislation to meet the costs of any damages awarded against them out of their own budget or by raising regulated loans. This could mean finding sums as high as £2.5 million for some of the obstetric claims. For this reason a concern was raised that the Trust Boards might try to recover part of the costs from the negligent employee. Although their vicarious liability would be difficult to avoid, it is possible in law to make a claim for contribution against the negligent employee. This was of particular concern to midwives. They practise in an area of high litigation costs – intrapartum care – and might have found that successful contribution claims would raise their professional indemnity insurance payments to an unacceptably high level. This problem has now receded for two reasons.

Following representation by the Royal College of Midwives in 1994, a Health Minister, Baroness Cumberlege, wrote an open letter in the *Midwives' Chronicle*. She said:

> 'Both health authorities and NHS trusts are responsible for the negligent acts and omissions of their midwife employees acting in the course of their employment.
>
> As improvements in practice occur through the implementation of *Changing Childbirth*, that position will remain the same.
>
> Insurance is desirable for any work done outside the NHS contract of employment, such as Good Samaritan acts in emergencies and providing midwifery services to friends and relatives.' [3]

Secondly, the Department of Health has proposed a new system to assist NHS Trusts to meet the litigation costs. Trusts will be able to pay into a central fund, from which pool of money claims will be met. It will be a voluntary arrangement but should spread the costs of major claims.

### The limits of vicarious liability

There are times when midwives express doubt about whether their employer will continue to accept vicarious liability and therefore indemnify them. The next section gives common examples that raise this question and discusses the position of the midwife in each.

#### Staying on duty

Joan has been looking after Sally since her admission in labour. Sally's labour is progressing well but she is not likely to deliver until an hour or so after Joan is due to go off duty. Joan discusses this with her manager who says she may not stay on duty because she will no longer be covered by the Trust if she works over the time when her shift ends. She has to explain this to Sally who is upset because they have become friendly over the past few hours. Joan hands over to a colleague and leaves.

This creates a lot of confusion and the reaction of the manager is not uncommon. Joan's employer cannot, in fact, avoid vicarious liability if she stays on duty. She is still carrying out work for her employer for which she is formally contracted; that is she is practising midwifery. Had she stayed on duty she would have been responding to the needs of her client. With the increasing emphasis on giving woman-centred care midwives will be expected to work more flexibly, and remaining on duty to deliver a woman is one way of fulfilling these obligations. It will not alter the legal relationship between the midwife and her employer.

#### Helping in an emergency

Sandra, a practising midwife, was shopping, when someone she knew ran up to her and asked her to come urgently into one of the shops. A woman was about to have a baby. They had called for the ambulance which hadn't yet arrived. Then they saw Sandra outside the shop. Sandra went in just in time to help the woman deliver a healthy baby boy.

In these emergency circumstances Sandra is not acting for her employer, but is performing a 'Samaritan act'. She cannot therefore expect to be indemnified by her employer. The law does not require Sandra to go to the assistance of the woman and she could have refused to help. It is not, however, clear what point of view would be taken by the UKCC on refusing to respond to a request to help and there is always the possibility that the Professional Conduct Committee would find such a refusal professional misconduct.

If Sandra decides to help the woman, then she will be personally accountable for her actions and, if Sandra were negligent, the woman could decide to sue her personally. If Sandra has no indemnity insurance, the woman is likely to be advised not to pursue a case as there would be little chance of receiving reasonable recompense. This would raise the ethical issue, however, of whether it is right for a professional to practise without offering insurance cover with the result that clients are denied an opportunity to seek proper redress if anything goes wrong.

Most professional associations and trade unions offer indemnity insurance which covers the midwife for 'Samaritan acts' as part of their subscription. Membership of such a scheme is advisable so that the midwife and her client are protected by insurance cover in these unexpected circumstances, and midwives should check with the association to which they belong that this cover is available to them.

This situation was obviously an emergency which was unconnected with Sandra's work. However, Sandra might have been a community midwife and when a neighbour called her in the middle of the night because his wife was about to deliver, she would respond to the call even though not on duty. In this case Sandra is likely to be seen as fulfilling her contractual obligations if the woman is booked for care by the maternity service that employs her.

### Delivering a friend

One of Caroline's closest friends asked her to deliver her baby. She was booked at a nearby hospital but not the one where Caroline worked. Caroline spoke to both her own manager/supervisor and the manager/supervisor of the other hospital, both of whom agreed that she might deliver her friend.

Most of the comments that applied to Sandra's case also apply here. Both Caroline's employer and the hospital where she intends to assist her friend are very unlikely to indemnify her, so Caroline will have to arrange this for herself. As long as she only very occasionally helps her friends, she will probably find that her subscription to a professional organization will include cover. She should nevertheless check that this is the case before saying 'yes' to her friend. It would be important if Caroline has no cover that she makes sure her friend knows this, putting it in writing. Her friend can then decide whether to still have Caroline's help. Although Caroline will remain liable for her actions even if not indemnified, without that cover her friend would have little chance of recovering significant levels of damages if something goes wrong. This raises more ethical than legal questions. Should a midwife offer professional services if she does not also offer indemnity cover in case things go wrong?

## Agreed protocols

Mr Jackson, a consultant obstetrician, sees the midwifery manager and gives her a protocol he has drawn up for the management of normal labour.

The manager looks at it and cannot agree with some of its requirements. She says that it would be better if the obstetricians and midwives could jointly agree a protocol and asks for a meeting. Mr Jackson says it is not necessary. He is the consultant obstetrician and therefore liable for what goes wrong. Thus he must dictate the policies of the unit. He added that if a midwife did not follow the protocol the hospital would not be vicariously liable in any subsequent malpractice case.

Mr Jackson is mistaken in two respects:

### Legal responsibility for a colleague

Midwives are held personally accountable for their actions by the UKCC, their professional body. This is also true in law and Mr Jackson's assertion that he is liable for the actions of the midwives is incorrect. The point is made in the case of *Rosen v. Edgar* (1986).

> Mrs Rosen had an operation for a bunion which was carried out by a senior registrar. She believed that the operation was performed negligently and sued the consultant in charge, a Mr Edgar.

The court held that Mr Edgar could not be held responsible for the actions of the registrar even though he was in charge of him. Except in the cases of actual supervision and training considered above an employee is not vicariously liable for the actions of another employee even if that person is junior to him and answerable to him.

If other cases of negligence are examined, it is clear that if a midwife is responsible it is her care which is criticized and not that of the consultant. In *Mitchell v. Hounslow and Spelthorne Health Authority* (1984) a midwife failed to give the correct first aid treatment when a woman had a prolapsed cord. It was held that this omission constituted a failure of what should have been normal standard practice in the circumstances by a competent midwife.

Because the midwife cannot avoid her own liability for the care she gives even if her employer is sued jointly with her, it is important that midwives are equally involved in drawing up the protocols for care and that these protocols are written in such a way that they still allow for individual clinical decision making if necessary.

### Acting outside the protocol

But what of the situation where a midwife finds herself unable to follow a protocol. Maybe she knows that research does not support it, or she may feel that her client's wishes override the protocol.

Mr Jackson was also wrong in suggesting that the hospital would not be responsible if a midwife acted outside the agreed protocol.

There are two cases, involving buses, *Limpus v. London General Omnibus Co.* (1862) and *Beard v. London General Omnibus Co.*

(1900) which illustrate the effect of explicit company policies on vicarious liability.

> In *Limpus*, a bus driver used his bus to obstruct another bus of a rival company even though there was a notice in the canteen expressly forbidding it. When his employer was sued for damage he had caused, the company claimed that he was working outside the terms of his employment because of the notice it had clearly displayed.
>
> In *Beard*, a bus driver had come to the end of his run. While he was temporarily away from the bus the conductor turned the bus around and, in doing so, caused some damage. Again the company claimed that it could not be vicariously liable as the conductor was working outside the terms of his contract.

In the first case, the court held that the driver was working within his contract even though he had disobeyed a company policy. The company could not avoid its liability even when the acts of its employee were negligent and in breach of its rules. The important point at issue was that he was employed to drive buses and that is what he was doing. But in the second case the conductor was not employed to drive the bus and the company was therefore able to claim that it was not liable for his actions.

Drawing an analogy with midwifery practice, the employer cannot escape liability even though the midwife does something which contravenes a hospital protocol if her actions still fall within the scope of midwifery practice, whereas the midwife who practises outside the normal definition of a midwife without the prior agreement of her employer will stand alone in any claim in negligence made against her.

The relationship between the autonomous clinical decisions of a midwife and health authority protocols was demonstrated in the recent events surrounding a waterbirth in East Hertfordshire Health Trust.

### Waterbirth – a problem of protocols

In December 1993 reports appeared in the press of the death of a baby born under water in Sweden and of the implication that two deaths in Bristol were related to the women spending some time in water in labour. The Royal College of Obstetricians issued a press statement condemning the practice as untested and in a number of press interviews suggested that delivery under water should not take place. There had been no randomized controlled trials on delivery under water but there were a number of audited cases and a national survey was being undertaken at the time. First findings would suggest that the procedure is as safe as any other way of giving birth.

As a result of the adverse press coverage a number of hospitals reissued their protocols banning birth under water. East Hertfordshire's policy allowed the woman to labour in water but not deliver in water.

One woman who was booked to have a homebirth told her midwife that she wished to labour and deliver under water. She hired a water pool. The midwife explained the existing protocol but the woman insisted on the delivery method of her choice. The midwife and a colleague successfully conducted the waterbirth. The NHS Trust however disciplined both midwives. There was an immediate outcry in the national press. The case did not go to court because there was no negligence but, if it had, the Trust would not have been able to avoid liability even though it had a policy banning waterbirth.

Through a personal communication with the Royal College of Midwives, the UKCC indicated its view on the matter. It drew attention to Rule 40 of the Midwives Rules and the responsibility laid upon the midwife to provide care to the mother and baby during the antenatal, intranatal and postnatal periods. It confirmed its position that the midwife should not refuse to continue to provide care even if in so doing she breaches her employer's policies. It went on to confirm the elements of good practice, which include giving the mother unbiased information upon which to base any decisions, discussing the problem with the Supervisor of Midwives and making clear records about the circumstances of the situation. It also set out the duty of the Supervisor of Midwives to ensure that local policies are easily available to midwives and that those policies should provide the midwife with support in all the settings in which she practises, including home births, so that the best possible arrangements can be made to care for the mother and baby.

In summary, protocols or guidelines for care can be very useful. They can be used for teaching purposes, as a guide for the newly appointed midwife and to remind all midwives of the correct framework for the care they give. A protocol should not be so inflexible that it stops a midwife from making clinical decisions in the best interests of her clients and both English law and the professional requirements of the UKCC would seem to uphold this point of view. Protocols are certainly not mechanisms by which one professional can dictate the work of another and they cannot be used by an employing authority to avoid its vicarious liability.

### Working on the 'bank'

> Anne is on the hospital's bank and usually works about twice a month. Her contract is with the hospital but only for duties as required.

A bank contract is a normal contract of employment even though it is for irregular hours of work. The employing authority is therefore still liable for the negligent actions of employees who hold these contracts so that Anne is in the same legal position as her colleagues who work full- or part-time.

### Working for an agency

> On the other hand, Alison has joined an agency. Like her friend she works
> about twice a month but it can be in different hospitals and occasionally she
> has been asked to cover some community clinics.

The situation for staff working for an agency is not quite so clear. Lord
Denning in his judgment in the case of *Roe* v. *Minister of Health*
(1954) stated that

> '. . . the hospital authorities are responsible for the whole of their staff,
> not only for the nurses and doctors, but also for the anaesthetists and
> surgeons. It does not matter whether they are permanent or tem-
> porary, resident or visiting, whole-time or part-time. The hospital
> authorities are responsible for all of them. The reason is because,
> even if they are not servants, they are the agents of the hospital to
> give the treatment. The only exception is the case of consultants or
> anaesthetists selected and employed by the patient himself.'

There are no cases directly concerned with agency midwives but it is
probable that the principle set by Lord Denning would apply, particularly where, as is beginning to happen, large hospitals are operating
their own free standing agency rather than using the commercial agency
sector. Midwives employed in this way are likely to be covered by the
hospital's liability. They would however be advised to check with the
hospital.

### Doing a locum

> Alison also helps out in the local independent midwives' practice. There are
> five of them and she usually covers them when they have holidays. They
> pay her a fee for the times she works for them.

There is no clarity in law about the liability in this case although any
direct employee of an independent midwife will have the same liability
cover as any other employee. Nelson-Jones and Burton [4] say in a
discussion of the liability of the general practitioner that

> 'it is unlikely that a general practitioner would be held liable for the
> negligent acts of a locum general practitioner unless it could be
> demonstrated that there was negligence in appointing the locum or
> failing to provide him with proper information.'

Anne would be well advised to have her own indemnity insurance cover
and the independent midwives' practice would also be advised to insist
on her having it.

### Working as a practice midwife

> Ruth has taken a job as a practice nurse. The general practitioner has asked her if she would also run the antenatal clinic, seeing some of the women and offering a limited domino delivery service. She has only just finished work as a midwife in the local hospital and attended a refresher course the year before. She therefore complies with the Midwives Rules but wonders whether she will be personally liable for potential malpractice and whether she needs to have personal professional indemnity.

If Ruth is employed by the general practitioner he will be vicariously liable for her actions. This is something that he should be fully aware of when employing Ruth as he may have to increase his medical practice insurance to cover her and to include the added responsibility of offering intrapartum care.

## Who can sue

Having looked at the extent of the midwife's liability and whether she is sued alone or whether for practical purposes the primary liability rests with someone else, this section will discuss the rights and opportunities that maternity clients have to sue their professional attendants.

Three things set this group of patients apart from other users of the health services:

(1) The fetus, although not legally alive, has limited rights of its own to seek redress for damage arising from negligence.

(2) The child has particular rights to legal aid that make it easier to use the legal system.

(3) There are two people involved in a maternity case, the mother and her child. Although highly unusual, there are occasions when the interests of each compete and the midwife or obstetrician may be forced to give optimal care to one at the expense of the other.

### The rights of women

This is straightforward. All women have the right to sue their attendants if they have possibly suffered as a result of negligence. They may find that their lawyer will advise against doing so because of the potential difficulty of proving a breach of the duty of care or establishing causation, or because the extent of the suffering would not attract sufficient monetary damages to warrant it.

Whilst physical damage such as paraplegia due to a faulty epidural will attract considerable damages to cover the cost of future care and loss of earnings, emotional damage attracts much less recompense. Lawyers will weigh up the level of potential damages against the complexity of the case when giving a woman advice.

A second limitation on a woman's opportunity to seek legal redress is the cost. A difficult legal case can lead to costs of as much as £250 000. Of course if the case is won these are met by the defendants but if the case is lost the woman must find the fees herself. It is this lottery which usually stops most patients from using the legal system, unless liability in principle is admitted early in the case.

In a case where the interests of the woman and baby compete, it is usually accepted that the woman's rights outweigh those of her unborn baby, but this will be discussed more fully in Chapter 6 on consent to treatment.

It is possible that a woman may be found to have contributed to the damage she has suffered and the court may use the doctrine of contributory negligence to reduce the compensation awarded on a percentage basis. The following cameos illustrate the point.

> Mrs Richards has had two previous postpartum haemorrhages and the midwife strongly advises her to have her baby in hospital. She nevertheless insists upon a home delivery. After the delivery she has a further haemorrhage, is transferred urgently to hospital and requires intensive care over a few weeks. She is left with Sheehan's Syndrome.

> Mrs Clarke has severe hypertension in pregnancy but refuses to go into hospital. She has an eclamptic fit at home and subsequently develops renal failure.

These are not actual legal cases because there has not been a midwifery case in England where contributory negligence has been used by the defence. The doctrine is well established in law however and it may well be that

● failure to answer questions when a history is being taken,
● failure to follow medical or midwifery advice,
● failure to comply with treatment schedules

could amount to contributory negligence which would diminish the liability of the professionals.

### The rights of the fetus/baby

Only living people have rights in law. Normally they cannot sue or be sued before they are born or after they are dead. Thus a case cannot be brought to redress loss of life for the victim, only for the loss suffered by his relatives. No damages will be payable for a baby born dead, or who dies shortly after birth, relating to his expectation of life, although the parents can sue for much reduced damages for their emotional suffering.

Until the mid 1970s this principle was absolute and applied equally to the fetus even if it could be proved that negligence in pregnancy caused an injury that would affect him for the rest of his life. Victims of the thalidomide disaster would not have been able to sue even if they could have proved all the elements of negligence. They were not alive when the women took the drug. All payments subsequently made were *ex gratia* and as a result of the public campaign on their behalf.

The thalidomide tragedy did, however, draw attention to the flaw in the law which barred these children from seeking legal recompense and as a result the Congenital Disabilities (Civil Liability) Act 1976 was passed.

### The Congenital Disabilities (Civil Liability) Act 1976

This Act established the right of the child to claim compensation for someone's negligent actions if he is disabled as a result of that negligence before his birth. The Act does not go so far as to establish a primary responsibility to the fetus but instead states the principle that if there is a duty of care to either parent and a breach of that duty of care harms the fetus, he will then have the right to sue. However, if there is no duty of care to the parents, the child has no right to sue for any harm done to him. Of course the midwife looking after a woman in pregnancy or labour has a duty of care in almost every circumstance towards her and therefore may be sued by the baby if he has been harmed by her actions or omissions before birth.

There are some exclusions in the Act. The child may not sue his mother unless she has been negligent whilst driving a car and is therefore covered by compulsory insurance. He may not sue if either or both parents knew of a pre-conception risk, although he may still sue his father if the father only knew of the risk and the mother did not.

The Act also states in section 5 the standard of professional care that is expected. It is almost the same as given in the *Bolam* case.

'The defendant is not answerable to the child for anything he did or omitted to do when responsible in a professional capacity for treating or advising the parent, if he took reasonable care having due regard to then received professional opinion applicable to the particular class of case, but this does not mean that he is unanswerable only because he departed from received opinion.'

### The baby's right to legal aid

Although the 1976 Act gave new rights to the fetus, it remained difficult for many families to sue for damages because of the high cost of litigation. Legal aid is only available to people on low income. A change in the legal aid regulations has made it easier for the baby to go to court as he may now be assessed for income purposes in his own right. As almost all babies have no income of their own this effectively means that they now have access to funds. A result of this change has been a rapid increase in obstetric litigation.

### Wrongful birth and wrongful life

Wrongful birth is the situation where a woman has had treatment to prevent her having another baby which fails, resulting in a pregnancy she did not want.

It has been established in law that she may claim for wrongful birth if after sterilization she subsequently has a baby. Damages are awarded that take account of the early costs of bringing up the child.

Wrongful life is the situation which arises when a child claims that it should never have been born. It would seem that by 1976 there were statutory provisions which would enable a child to sue for wrongful life. The Abortion Act 1967 allowed a doctor to assist a woman to have an abortion as long as certain legal principles were adhered to and the Congenital Disabilities (Civil Liability) Act 1976 gave the fetus a limited right to sue if it was harmed by someone's negligence.

The case of *Mckay* v. *Essex Area Health Authority* (1985), was brought in the name of a child claiming that she had been wrongfully born.

> Mrs Mckay was tested antenatally for rubella and told that she had not been infected in the pregnancy. She subsequently gave birth to a daughter who was severely handicapped as a result of rubella infection. The child alleged that she should not have been born at all.

It was held that there could be no duty towards the fetus to cause its death. The principle of wrongful life was rejected as contrary to public policy.

## Time limits for litigation

People do not have an unlimited time to take legal action. The Limitation Act 1980 normally requires that an action should be commenced within three years of the alleged negligence. This may be extended to six years where the action is not related to personal injury. After that the action is time-barred.

There are, however, important exceptions to this that relate to maternity care.

## Date of knowledge

Imagine a situation where someone has been taking a prescribed drug for many years and develops side effects. Perhaps some time afterwards he learns that his problems were probably caused by the drug he had been taking. Many years may have elapsed from first being prescribed the drug. If the courts applied the three year ruling to the time when he first had treatment he would be time-barred. This would be a clear injustice. The Limitation Act 1980 allows for this situation in that it permits a case to be brought within three years from the plaintiff's presumed knowledge of potential negligence.

## Children and persons of unsound mind

In maternity care there are two particular circumstances which considerably extend the usual time limit.

A child is not deemed able to have knowledge of the potential cause of his injury until he has reached 18. Time starts to run against him from that point. He therefore may start an action at any time up to his twenty-first birthday.

If a person is of unsound mind within the meaning of the Mental Health Act 1983 (that is, he is incapable of running his own affairs and this includes arrested or incomplete development of mind), time will not run out for him. If his condition persists, an action may be brought in his name at any time during his lifetime. This would certainly apply to babies who are brain damaged.

# A case of negligence – what happens

Chapter 1 briefly described the legal process once a plaintiff issues a writ to the point where a trial takes place. But what happens to the midwife who may be involved?

## Writing up notes

It is often possible to anticipate clinical circumstances which may lead to a civil action. The difficult delivery where the baby needs resuscitation; the baby who has neonatal convulsions; the unexpected stillbirth. Although staff may believe that their care has been of an acceptable standard and that their relationship with the mother has been good, this is no guarantee that the parents will not seek legal redress if their baby is brain damaged.

It is always better to assume that this may be the case and as soon as possible after the event write extra full notes recording the events and main elements of the care given to the woman and her baby. This should be discussed with the supervisor of midwives and it may also be useful to hold a case conference to discuss the management of the case in detail.

### Writing a statement

If the parents approach a solicitor he will give them initial advice on the merits of the case. He is then very likely to write to the hospital indicating that his clients are contemplating a legal action. He will set out the reasons for this. This letter will be referred to the hospital's legal advisers and shortly afterwards each of the clinical staff involved in the care will be contacted and asked to write a statement about their part in it. This request will not necessarily be confined to the primary carer in the case but may be directed to everyone whose signatures appear in the case notes during the time relevant to the complaint.

This first statement is of great importance. It will enable the employer's legal advisers to assess the extent of their liability and where their case has weaknesses. It will eventually be handed to the plaintiff's lawyers.

It must be accurately written and reflect where possible the reasons for any decision-making that took place. Yet the request may come months or even years after the events took place. Any midwife who is asked to write a statement should therefore seek help both from her employers and, if possible, from outside. Most trade unions and professional organizations offer support for statement writing and the midwife should make contact with her representative. Where the midwife's role in the case was minimal, assistance may be given over the telephone or by letter. If, however, the midwife is directly involved in the events leading to the alleged injury, it may be necessary for her to meet her representative.

Help will also be available from the employer. This is a situation, unlike that arising from a disciplinary action, where the interests of the employer and employee are the same. The employer will be anxious to avoid expensive claims if there has clearly been no negligence. If there has been, it usually in the interests of the employer to recognize this and pursue a settlement out of court. It will at the least save the huge legal expenses that accompany these actions. If the midwife has been negligent it will probably, in the long run, not be helpful to her to be uncooperative in any enquiry arising from potential litigation.

One source of help that the employer can offer, will be their legal advisers. It may appear to be daunting to meet with lawyers but they can often clarify the legal position and give advice on how best to write the statement. An interview with the legal advisers can be attended also by the midwife's representative and in this way a statement can be jointly drawn up.

Before a statement is finalized, it can go through a number of drafts.

Apart from making sure that all available help is obtained, there are other principles which should be followed.

(1) Never write a statement without the case notes to refer to.

(2) Always ask for a copy of the original complaint. It is impossible to write a statement answering specific allegations without knowing exactly what they are. It is surprising how many times midwives are asked to write about their management of a case without this vital information. If it is not forthcoming, the representative should be asked to get it.

(3) Write factually. The case notes will be available to the plaintiff's lawyers so discrepancies between the statement and the notes will be spotted quickly.

(4) Additional information can be given, for example why decisions were made or not made, even though this may not appear in the notes, but only if it is accurately remembered. If the case gets to court the plaintiff's lawyers will undoubtedly question the facts of the statement, particularly if they are not contained in the case notes. If recollection is hazy it may be best to leave the matter out. This should be discussed with both the legal advisers and professional representative.

(5) Do not include 'hearsay'. Only include those events with which you were directly involved and report only those things you were personally told about, identifying the source of information.

(6) Do not sign the final statement until completely satisfied with the accuracy of its contents. Sometimes after the first interview with the lawyers they re-write the statement. They do not know the technical details of midwifery care and can get it wrong. Do not be afraid to discuss this with them and get them to amend it.

(7) Keep a copy.

## After the statement stage

Writing and signing a statement may be the last that a midwife will hear of a case. The notes and statements will be sent to the plaintiff's lawyers and the long process of negotiation with them will begin. Sometimes it will be apparent that there is no case to answer, in others the negligence is obvious. In either case the lawyers will try for settlement. Almost all cases are ended in this way. A very few however do come to trial, especially when the facts of the case are in dispute or when there is no agreement about the level of damages to be awarded.

If a case is likely to come to court, the solicitors should meet with all their witnesses to discuss the questions they are going to be asked and the general content of the answers. The solicitors will also try to anticipate the questions that the plaintiff's lawyers may ask and will discuss the possible answers. This pre-hearing preparation is very important.

Again it may be useful to have a representative there who can take notes and go over some of the discussions afterwards. The situation is not very different from that of a woman being given difficult information by a consultant and the midwife spending some time afterwards clarifying it and answering any further queries.

### The hearing

At the trial the case is invariably brought primarily against the employer rather than the practitioner. The employer will therefore be represented and will call all the involved staff as witnesses. A witness may not be represented in court but, as this can be a very upsetting experience, professional organizations usually offer a support service, providing one of their stewards or officers to stay with a midwife during the hearing.

As a witness, the midwife will only be in the court for the duration of her evidence. She will be questioned by the lawyers for the defence first and then cross-examined by the plaintiff's lawyers. Obviously the second set of questions will be more difficult that the first. Again some rules will help.

(1) Be factual. Just as when writing the statement, any deviation from the facts will be quickly noted and the plaintiff's barrister could exploit this with further questions to discredit your evidence.

(2) Do not be led into conjecture unless you are very confident that your opinion would be acceptable to 'the ordinary skilled practitioner'.

(3) Always check that you fully understand the questions. You can ask for clarification. One of the responsibilities of the judge is to ensure that witnesses understand all they are being asked. If the questions are very obscure you should say so and ask for help interpreting them.

(4) If you need to see evidence such as the case notes to refresh your memory, ask to see them. Being a witness is not an examination and you are not expected to have memorized the facts of the case.

(5) The events of the case may have happened some years before. If you do not remember something, say so. Do not try to dredge up inaccurate facts from a long time ago.

(6) If you did make mistakes in the management of the case, do not try to justify them unreasonably. Before the hearing you should care-

fully discuss this with your employer's lawyers and consider with them how to present these in court.

(7) Stay calm. If you get flustered, you may not answer questions as well as you might. Remember that it is the job of the plaintiff's barrister to show up your actions in the worst possible light. Do not get angry. Just remember that your reasoned answers are the best way to refute this.

### After the trial

The trial is almost certainly the last time that the practitioner will be directly involved in any proceedings. It is possible for the case to be referred to the Court of Appeal and on to the House of Lords (remember the case of *Whitehouse* v. *Jordon* (1981)). These are not new trials. The judges look only at the transcripts of the cases and the submitted evidence when coming to their opinion. Witnesses are not called.

### Cases of alleged malpractice – the midwife manager's role

Whenever an allegation of malpractice is made involving midwives, the manager has a role to play. It is usually the midwife manager who will make first contact with the midwife and will then form the link between her and the legal advisers and general management. The midwife is likely to be very upset that a complaint has been made and anxious about the process. Although the manager has the responsibility to make sure that statements are obtained, she can also offer support and informal counselling to the midwife, including a reminder that she should contact her professional organization for outside, unbiased help.

The manager should also assist in obtaining the clinical notes and a copy of the complaint and may also need to arrange for meeting rooms and time away off duty so that the midwife can discuss the case with her representative. The local steward may be asked to give some direct support, especially if the midwife has to go to court, and the steward should be given time off for this duty.

The manager may also be required to act as co-ordinator if there is more than one discipline involved. Because of her possible pivotal role in the process, she should be certain of what is likely to happen and, if necessary, should also arrange to see the legal advisers so they can tell her how the case might proceed.

Sometimes a case depends on evidence of staffing levels and other related management procedures, such as the way in which a theatre is obtained for caesarean section. In these circumstances the manager may also be required to give a statement and appear as a witness as part of the employer's case.

### The midwife as expert witness

The standard of care that the courts use is that of the 'ordinary skilled practitioner'. To determine this both sides in a case use expert witnesses and midwives are used where a midwife's care is in question.

If a midwife is asked to act as a witness it will usually be by recommendation to the solicitor. In the first instance the request will usually be to look at the facts of the clinical care in relation to the complaint and to give an adjudication in writing about whether the standard of care was wanting. The request to act as a witness can come from either side in a dispute, but it is the responsibility of the witness to give impartial evidence based on her clinical knowledge. At this early stage her advice may be invaluable to the parties in deciding whether to settle or go to court.

If the case goes to trial, the expert witness may be called to give evidence. When first approached to act as witness the midwife should indicate whether she is willing to give evidence at court. It is not helpful for the lawyers to have to change a witness part way through a case.

If asked to act as a witness, the midwife should also think carefully about whether she is properly qualified to do so. If the events occurred some time ago, the case will be judged on the standards prevailing at the time. If the midwife was not practising at the time, or was newly qualified, she should tell the lawyers this so they can assess whether she can speak with authority on the points raised by the case.

Being an expert witness can be difficult. It requires a detailed assessment of the case, the production of a report and a possible court appearance. It does attract a fee.

## AVOIDING LITIGATION

The increase in obstetric litigation and the rising costs associated with legal fees and awards for damages have resulted in a debate within the professions about how to curtail such costs in the future. Concern is also being expressed about the effect that the litigation threat can have upon the clinical care offered and the willingness of professionals to practise in 'high risk' specialties. The experience in the United States, where it is somewhat easier for people to go to court than in the UK, suggests evidence of adverse outcomes of rising litigation.

- Doctors have tended to practise defensively, doing tests and treatments that were not necessary so that they could not be accused later of not offering all possible care. The high rate of caesarean section could be explained in part by this approach.

- The level of malpractice insurance rose considerably so that in some States it costs the individual obstetrician $40 000 a year. This has led many obstetricians to stop practising so that women are now unable to get the services of an obstetrician.

The inter-professional debates have focused on two main solutions, a reform of the compensation system and the adoption of a risk management approach to clinical care.

## Reforming the compensation system

The current system in the UK depends upon the plaintiff proving that someone has been at fault in order to get compensation. The advantage of such a system is that the negligence of a named health care professional is made explicit and this can act as a powerful mechanism for maintaining professional standards.

However, the need to prove fault can polarize the two sides in a case, with both relying heavily on expensive expert witnesses and prolonged legal argument to prove or disprove alleged facts. Pre-hearing discussions between the lawyers can be very protracted, contributing to an increase in costs. All of this can delay the time of the financial settlement by years even though the needs of the disabled person may be very immediate.

The system can also be a 'lottery' for the plaintiff with no guarantee that he will receive compensation. Compensation can be more dependent upon the skills of his lawyers than upon his need for financial help and whether or not it is paid may not be linked to his actual needs. Remember the case of *Whitehouse* v. *Jordon* (1981). Stuart Whitehouse was 11 years old when the final judgment was made in the House of Lords and in the end he had no compensation. Yet he was severely brain damaged and had great needs that were not being met.

One solution to this dilemma is to abolish the requirement to prove fault in order to receive financial recompense and introduce 'no fault compensation'. This system, which was introduced in Sweden and New Zealand, depends instead upon proving that there has been a medical accident for which compensation will be paid. Rather than the professionals being directly responsible for paying the compensation (through their indemnity insurance schemes), a national fund was set up from which the compensation would be paid.

Many professionals and their organizations, including the British Medical Association have argued for the introduction of such a system in order that:

- cases can be decided more quickly;
- there can be more certainty in the outcome of a case for the plaintiff; and
- the professional would be able to practise without the threat of litigation.

There are also arguments against the introduction of no fault compensation. Indeed a committee which looked at whether to introduce the system, rejected it on the grounds that it would be prohibitively expensive and that there may be just as much delay and uncertainty for the plaintiff. It would simply substitute proof of medical accident for proof of fault.

Also there may be less pressure upon the professionals to maintain their standards of practice if they were not in danger of being identified as personally at fault. Indeed this is the current position of the organization, Action for the Victims of Medical Accidents.

The arguments against no fault compensation have increased since both of the countries who originally introduced the scheme are now modifying it. Although standards of care do not seem to have dropped since its introduction, both are seeking radical change because the system has proved very expensive and victims are not finding it easy to prove medical accident any more than it was easy to prove medical fault. It also excludes from any compensation those who cannot prove accident, just as such victims are excluded in the UK if they cannot prove fault, even though their needs may be just as great as those of others who can.

## A risk management approach

If changing the legal system will not bring about improvements to the system of recompense, then the medical and midwifery professions should examine ways of minimizing the danger of litigation whilst still protecting the interests of their clients. The principle of risk management first gained ground in the United States and is being increasingly adopted in the UK.

A study on the incidence of adverse events and negligence in hospitalized patients was conducted by Harvard University in 1984 [5]. It was not confined to any special group so does not reflect obstetric care specifically. It found that there was a substantial amount of injury to patients from medical management and many of the injuries were the result of sub-standard care.

No study has been conducted into obstetric cases but based upon these findings the Beth Israel Hospital in Boston introduced a very structured approach to clinical care.

- It first arranged a series of multi-disciplinary conferences and from these developed clinical protocols based on up-to-date research knowledge.

- It then instituted a systematic review of clinical notes to check whether the protocols had been adhered to.

- If they were not followed the explanation for not following them had to be clearly stated in the notes.

- If it was not, the clinician, whether doctor or midwife, was interviewed to discover why.

- If the reason was not satisfactory, this could lead to some form of sanction.

This may sound very draconian and the obstetric consultant has admitted that it has led to a reduction in clinical freedom. But the medical negligence cases have fallen since the system was introduced, the level of payment for damages has been reduced and with it the level of professional indemnity premiums for the staff.

Risk management is about following a structured approach to reduce identifiable risk before problems arise, rather than dealing with them afterwards. A simple framework can be followed:

(1) Agree standards of care based upon current research and write clinical guidelines based upon these.

(2) Take particular care over those areas of care which are most likely to attract litigation. In a booklet for the Royal College of Midwives [6], six main concerns in midwifery practice are listed:

    (a) failure to respond appropriately to meconium staining of amniotic liquor,

    (b) failure to respond appropriately to abnormalities in CTG traces,

    (c) delay in summoning medical assistance,

    (d) differences of opinion with regard to how bad things have to be before one intervenes,

    (e) an incomplete evidential picture caused by inadequate record keeping especially in relation to decisions to 'wait and see', and

    (f) failure to follow up bad outcomes and establish a full labour record or to identify paediatric evidence relevant to causation.

(3) Start a systematic and frequent review of clinical notes checking the care given against the agreed clinical guidelines and checking notes for completeness.

(4) Start a systematic case discussion process to highlight both difficult and apparently normal cases which should be picked at random.

(5) Introduce a continuous training programme to cover areas of concern such as CTG interpretation.

(6) Ensure an immediate case conference on all adverse outcomes, to include the preparation of statements about these.

This may sound prescriptive and contrary to the principles of clinical freedom. However, if it is properly done in a supportive atmosphere and where all disciplines are equally involved the result can be a considerable raising of standards.

It cannot be stressed strongly enough that the proper maintenance of clinical records is central to proving the facts surrounding alleged malpractice and this is discussed in detail in Chapter 7 on record keeping.

# OTHER WAYS OF SEEKING REDRESS

## The complaints procedure

The Hospital Complaints Procedure Act 1985 and the National Health Service and Community Care Act 1990 require the Secretary of State to issue guidance on the process for handling complaints and this is contained in Health Circular, HC(88)37. This is due for amendment following the report of the Wilson Committee [7] which had been reviewing the NHS complaints procedure. The proper application of the complaints procedure is not likely to deflect parents from making a legal claim if their case is serious. There is, however, some evidence that they would not seek legal redress for trivial matters if their initial complaint was sensitively handled.

The Circular sets out the following requirements:

- Each health authority must designate a senior officer to be responsible for complaints.

- It must be recognized that all patients to have the right to complain or a close relative may do so on their behalf if they are unable to do so.

- Complaints must be dealt with quickly and sensitively.

- Complaints must be monitored.

Like any other circumstance when a woman or her family choose to complain, a complaint under the procedure can be very upsetting for the midwife concerned. She should co-operate with the managers in trying to resolve the complaint but should also contact her professional association so that she can receive unbiased support.

## The Health Service Commissioner

The Health Service Commissioners Act 1993 provides for the appointment of a Health Service Commissioner for England and one for Wales. The Commissioner may investigate a complaint about health authority services or maladministration if a complainant is not satisfied with the outcome of the authority's own investigation of the complaint. He may not deal with complaints about clinical decisions. Many of the applications to the Commissioner are about failures and delays in dealing with complaints.

## The Community Health Council

Community Health Councils were first set up in 1974 and the current statutory provision for them is contained in the National Health Service Act 1977. It is the duty of the Community Health Council to protect the interests of the public in its district. It acts as a 'watchdog' by monitoring actions and plans of the local health services. It can help people who are dissatisfied with the service they have received by giving them advice on how to complain but usually does not help people to complain.

## SUMMARY

The midwife is accountable for her practice and the standards she should maintain.

Allegations and complaints may be reported to the UKCC which will decide whether or not she has been guilty of professional misconduct.

If her negligent action has injured her client, either the woman or the baby, her employing authority may be vicariously liable for her actions but, where she is not employed, she may be found to be personally liable in law.

A woman may also use the hospital complaints procedure if she is unhappy about her care, and if her complaint is not satisfactorily dealt with she may ask the Health Service Commissioner to investigate it.

These difficult circumstances can be avoided by adopting a risk management approach to try to ensure that practitioners meet required standards, that there is a formal system of auditing the care given and that records of care are carefully made.

If involved in any complaint, the midwife should seek support from her professional organization or trade union.

## FURTHER ACTION

- Discuss how you and your colleagues can adopt risk management in your unit/service/practice.

- Ask the complaints officer to talk to you and your colleagues about how complaints are investigated and about the results of the monitoring procedures.

- Contact the Health Service Commissioner's office, Church House, Great Smith Street, London SWIP 3B (071–276 3000), and invite a representative to speak in a local study day.

# REFERENCES

1. United Kingdom Central Council for Nursing, Midwifery and Health Visiting. *Complaints about Professional Conduct*. London, UKCC, 1993.
2. Acheson, Sir D. Are Obstetrics and Midwifery Doomed? The Sir Wiliam Powell Memorial Lecture. *The Midwives' Chronicle*, **104**, (1241) June 1991, pp 158–66.
3. Baroness Cumberlege. Open letter to Midwives. *The Midwives' Chronicle*, **107** (1275) p. 124.
4. Nelson-Jones, R. and Burton. F. Medical Negligence and Case Law. London, Fourmat Publishing, 1990.
5. Bennen, T.A., Leape. L.L., Laird N.M. et al, Incidence of Adverse Effects and Negligence in Hospitalised Patients: Results of the Harvard Medical Practice. *New England Jnl of Med.*, **324** (6) Feb 7th 1991.
6. Mason, D. Edwards, P. and Capstick, B. *Litigation: a risk management guide for midwives*. London, Royal College of Midwives, 1993.
7. Review Committee on NHS Complaints Procedures (Wilson Committee). *Being Heard: The Report of a Review Committee on NHS Complaints Procedures*. Leeds, DoH, 1994.

# Chapter 6
# Consent to Treatment

## GENERAL LEGAL PRINCIPLES

All health care professionals know about formal written consent to treatment. In some form or another written consent has always been used prior to surgery or other major invasive medical treatments. But consent to treatment is legally far more complex than just getting the signature of a willing patient.

In an American case, *Schloendorff* v. *Society of the New York Hospital* (1914) the judge made the basic point:

'Every human being of adult years and sound mind has a right to determine what shall be done with his own body.'

If this right is removed and something is done without consent, whether it is major surgery or a simple test such as taking a blood pressure, then the professional can be held to have committed battery upon the patient.

Even if consent seems to have been obtained, if proper information has not been given to help the patient to decide what to do, the courts may find that the professional has been negligent in the giving of information or advice.

There are therefore two areas of law concerned with obtaining consent, battery in carrying out the treatment without consent and negligence in failing to give required advice for informed consent.

## Battery and consent

This is both a criminal and civil offence and is the intentional or reckless unlawful application of force against another person. Even to touch someone without consent could be defined as the civil offence of trespass to the person. Should a health care professional be confronted with either of these claims the most widely used defence would be that the person consented to the treatment.

Although written consent is obtained for major invasive treatment it would be impossible to obtain it every time a treatment or test was performed. But because of the nature of consent this is not necessary because consent can be either implied or expressly given.

### Implied consent

Consent is implied where the actions of people would imply that they do not object to what is to be done to them. This is the commonest form of consent to treatment and applies to almost all midwifery and nursing care.

> The midwife says she is going to take a woman's blood pressure, or even approaches the woman with the sphygmomanometer without saying a word, and the woman rolls up the sleeve of her jumper.

Neither will have spoken but the action of the woman clearly implies that she has no objection to the test.

There is no need to record that implied consent was given. The recording of the blood pressure in the notes would normally be sufficient to imply that it was done with consent.

### Express consent

Consent can, however, be expressly obtained either in writing or verbally. It usual and very wise to obtain consent in writing for all planned invasive treatment, hence the use of the standard consent to treatment form.

There may be occasions however where written consent cannot be obtained when a procedure is invasive, even when the patient is completely able to make a rational decision about treatment.

> A midwife is delivering a baby, the head is on the perineum and she decides an episiotomy is necessary. It is an invasive surgical operation for which she must obtain consent. The woman is 'of sound mind' and able to give consent but it is clearly not possible to get consent in writing.

Express consent, given verbally should be obtained.

### The legal position

The law sees no difference in the importance of these ways of obtaining consent, the only difference being in the ease of proving that consent has been obtained.

However, getting the courts to accept that battery has occurred is not easy. Most cases that have been brought have claimed not only that consent was not obtained but also that insufficient information was given to enable any consent to be valid. These will be discussed further in the section on giving information, but most of the judgments have not accepted a claim of battery except in the circumstance where consent has been expressly withheld. An example is *Cull v. Butler and Another* (1932).

> A woman agreed to curettage but expressly stated that she did not want a hysterectomy. Her uterus was removed and she sued the surgeon and the hospital.

It was held that the hospital was in negligent breach of contract with the patient *and* that the surgeon had trespassed against her person.

Liability has also been found in cases where the treatment given has considerably exceeded that which the patient agreed to. Performing sterilization (unconsented) at the same time as doing caesarean section or giving a blood transfusion to a Jehovah's Witness are both situations which have come to court and where the court supported the patient's argument. (*Hamilton* v. *Birmingham Regional Hospital Board* (1969)).

### Treatment when consent cannot be obtained

There are times when treatment must be given and yet the person is unable to give consent, for example the unconscious patient needing surgery or the woman with eclampsia who must have urgent treatment and be delivered. Here medical and midwifery staff can use the defence of 'necessity' to protect them from legal action.

These two examples are very straightforward. But there are many other circumstances where the decision on whether the person is of sound mind is a question of degree and clinical judgment.

Take the following case study:

> Angela has been looking after Carol who is in labour. She had pethidine 45 minutes ago. Her membranes rupture and the liquor is heavily contaminated with meconium. Angela is preparing to examine Carol vaginally when she notices that the CTG tracing is showing sudden and severe type two dips. She rings immediately for the consultant. On vaginal examination the cervix is only 6cm dilated. The consultant decides upon an immediate caesarean section. Carol is very sedated as a result of having the pethidine. She is able to sign a consent form but both Angela and the consultant are not sure whether she has understood the implications of the operation and the general anaesthetic.

It would be very difficult for the law to develop any hard and fast principles to guide staff in these circumstances. It would expect the clinical decision to be made in all good faith and that the consultant would follow a course of action that a body of ordinary skilled practitioners would also follow. It would expect to see evidence that the professional has positively assessed the competence of the woman to give consent.

In this case the obstetrician should clearly ask himself: 'is Carol able to understand the decision I am asking her to make and the implications of that decision which I am explaining to her?'. If the answer is 'yes', then Carol's decision on her treatment must be followed. If the answer is 'no, Carol is so sedated that she does not understand the implications of the situation, but she nevertheless needs to have a caesarean section' then the treatment can go ahead. If it is subsequently questioned in court the defence of necessity can then be used.

This test for competence should be applied in all cases where there is doubt about the woman's ability to understand the treatment that is being advised. It will be of no use if it cannot be proved so it is of great importance that the assessment of competence is clearly indicated in the medical record.

There are two other circumstances in which judgment may be impaired so that obtaining consent may be more problematical: consent obtained from a minor and from someone who is mentally impaired.

## Consent by minors

Adulthood is reached in the UK at the age of 18 and the law accepts the absolute right of a person over that age and of sound mind to decide what happens to his body.

The Family Law Reform Act 1969 gives the statutory right to all young people between the ages of 16 and 18 to decide on whether to have medical treatment or not.

### Gillick

The rights of children below that age to give consent were decided by a House of Lords decision in the case of *Gillick* v. *West Norfolk and Wisbech Area Health Authority* (1986).

> Mrs Gillick had five daughters under the age of 16. In 1985 the Department of Health and Social Security issued a circular saying that it would be lawful for a doctor to prescribe contraceptives to a girl under 16 on her consent alone provided he acted in good faith. He could do this in exceptional circumstances without the consent of the parents and without informing them. Mrs Gillick challenged this circular.

A decision of the House of Lords confirmed the contents of the circular. They held that a girl under 16 did not lack the legal capacity to give consent on grounds of age only. Lord Fraser summed up the decision thus:

'It seems to me verging on the absurd to suggest that a girl or boy aged 15 could not effectively consent, for example, to have a medical examination of some trivial injury to his body or even to have his arm set. Of course the consent of the parents should normally be asked, but they may not be immediately available . . .'

Lord Scarman added

'Parental right yields to the child's right to make his own decisions when he reaches a sufficient understanding and intelligence to be capable of making up his own mind on the matter requiring decision . . .'

Of course the young child cannot understand the implications of medical treatment, but the *Gillick* judgment rejects age as an impediment to consent and suggests that the rule should be sufficient understanding. Users of maternity care, even the very young, have reached puberty so the decision about whether they may give consent is usually not difficult. Also it will be the very rare occasion that a parent is not available or refuses treatment for the child.

In these circumstances, either the young woman's own consent should be obtained, or, as a last resort, the treatment may be considered using the doctrine of necessity. Finally, if there is time to do so, the hospital may seek to make the child a ward of court and get the court's permission to carry out treatment.

### Wardship

Wardship may be the best course of action where the parent is actively opposing treatment rather than not being present to consent.

Religious conviction can sometimes lead parents to withhold consent for the necessary treatment of their children. In the case of *Re P (a minor)* (1981), the girl's father, a Seventh Day Adventist, opposed the termination of his 15-year old daughter's second pregnancy. She was at the time in the care of Lewisham Borough Council. The Council made her a ward of court and sought the court's permission for termination. It was granted and, in addition, the court confirmed its view that the Council had acted properly.

### Consent when the person is mentally impaired

Where emergency treatment is required, the usual defence of necessity can be relied upon when the patient is mentally impaired. There are now two cases that have determined the position regarding consent to other less urgent and long term treatments that may be necessary. In *Re B (a minor)* (1988) the facts were as follows

> A 17-year old in the care of Sutherland Borough Council was made a ward of court and the court asked to give consent to sterilization. Her mental capacity was of a six-year old. She was incapable of understanding the relationship between sexual intercourse and pregnancy and incapable of understanding contraception, but she was showing signs of sexual awareness by making sexual approaches to male staff and other patients.

Leave was given to perform the operation and the Court of Appeal and the House of Lords upheld the decision. Because B was a minor, a court could give consent on her behalf.

However, in a second and similar case, the woman was 36-years old.

Under the Mental Health Act 1983 there is no statutory power for the courts to give or withhold consent to treatment of an adult, even though the adult is incompetent in the meaning of the Act. The facts in *F* v. *West Berkshire Health Authority* (1989) were as follows:

> F was a 36-year old woman with a mental capacity of about four. She had started a sexual relationship with another patient but in the view of the doctors it would not be in her best interests to become pregnant. Her mother sought a declaration that it would not be unlawful to perform a sterilization.

The case was decided in the House of Lords where it was said that the courts could not consent to treatment for an adult but that a court could declare the lawfulness of a proposed operation. To be lawful, even though without consent;

- the treatment should be in the best interests of the patient; and
- the doctor must act in accordance with a responsible and competent body of medical opinion.

This last sentence refers back to the principles first given in the *Bolam* case.

Lord Bridge said in his judgment:

> 'It would be intolerable for members of the medical, nursing and other professions devoted to the care of the sick that, in caring for those lacking the capacity to consent to treatment, they should be put in the dilemma that, if they administer the treatment which they believe to be in the patient's best interest, acting with due skill and care, they run the risk of being held guilty of trespass to the person, but if they

withhold that treatment they may be in breach of a duty of care owed to the patient.'

This judgment does not open the way to uncontrolled, unconsented treatment of people who are mentally impaired. It does, however, allow the usual treatments to be performed, including emergency treatment. A court declaration on the lawfulness of untoward and serious treatment such as sterilization will probably still be needed in the future.

### Consent by a woman's husband or partner

In the case of Carol, given earlier in this chapter, it would be good clinical practice to discuss the need for the operation with Carol's husband or partner, or indeed any other close relative who may be with her in labour. However the consent of a husband or partner is not recognized or needed in law.

In the case of a woman's sterilization, for example, it now less common for the obstetrician to demand the signature of the woman's husband. Legally, no such consent has ever been required. It could be argued strongly that both legally and ethically it would be wrong to withhold a treatment which a woman wants and has consented to because another person, even her husband, disagrees.

## Giving information and advice

It is not sufficient to get consent to a treatment, whether in writing or not. The practitioner must also be able to show that information was given to help the patient to make an informed decision.

There is no doctrine of informed consent in English law. In the United States, where the doctrine exists, the medical practitioner or nurse must give a patient information that the patient would, if asked, say he would need to make a decision. The information given should therefore cover most, if not all, the potential dangers of the procedure, so that the patient can weigh these up against the advantages of the treatment.

The standard expected in Britain was defined in a leading case, *Sidaway* v. *Board of Governors of Bethlem Royal Hospital and the Maudsley Hospital and Others* (1985).

> Mrs Sidaway had persistent pain in her arm and shoulder. She had a laminectomy to free a nerve but during the operation her spinal cord was damaged and she was left with severe disability. She sued, claiming that the surgeon had been negligent in not informing her of the possibility of spinal cord damage. The surgeon had told her there was a small risk of disturbing a nerve root but had not indicated there was a danger of paralysis. He did not want to frighten her for what was a less than one per cent risk.

The case went to the House of Lords where the judgment was made in favour of the defendants. Mrs Sidaway lost the case.

As with so many of the other similar decisions, the *Bolam* test was used. A number of medical witnesses, accepted as a responsible body of medical opinion, agreed they would have given the same information as Mrs Sidaway's surgeon.

The guiding principle therefore in the UK is professional consensus about what should be communicated to the patient.

## Woman's consent and fetal rights

So far this chapter has stressed that a person who has reached adulthood and is of sound mind can consent or withhold consent to treatment and that people have a right to determine what happens to their own body.

The pregnant woman presents a different situation from the normal. She is carrying a fetus and treatments she either has or refuses to have could damage her unborn child.

The law has been very clear in the past on the status of the fetus. It does not exist and therefore cannot have rights in law.

This has been very carefully modified for negligence actions by the Congenital Disabilities (Civil Liability) Act 1976, but even this Act protects the relationship between woman and fetus, giving protection to the woman over that of the child as the primary duty of care is still to the mother. There is no liability towards the fetus if there is no duty of care to the woman and where there is conflict the mother's interests will still prevail under the Act.

There have been some past cases in the UK which have attempted to make the rights of the fetus paramount such as the case known as *Re F (in utero)* (1988).

> There was an attempt to make an unborn child a ward of court because there was no guarantee that its mother, a drug addict, would stay in one place and attend for necessary antenatal care. The wardship order may have opened the possibility of detaining the woman and forcing her to have treatments for the sake of the fetus.

The Court of Appeal judges unanimously rejected the application.

In the United States there have been a few notorious cases where women have been forced to have a caesarean section against their express wishes. The facts of *Re AC* (1990) are particularly distressing.

> AC was a young woman who had had cancer and was pregnant. The cancer reappeared and the hospital withheld treatment to protect the health of the unborn child. It obtained a declaration that it could perform a

caesarean section to save the life of the child even though AC would probably not survive it. AC refused to have the operation and appealed against the declaration. She failed and the operation was performed. Both she and the baby died.

There was a public outcry and her estate sued the hospital. The Appeal Court found the declaration to be unsafe. It said that such an intervention should virtually never be justified and it was not justified in this case. Even where the mother is dying she should, if of sound mind, be able to grant or withhold consent. As a result of this case the American Medical Association and the American College of Obstetricians and Gynaecologists have accepted that no pregnant woman should be coerced into any treatment against her will.

This should have settled the matter, but the case of *Re S* (1992) is inconsistent with this position. This is an extremely important English case which all midwives should be aware of as it again challenges the rights of the pregnant woman.

> A 30-year old woman was in labour. She was six days overdue and had ruptured membranes. The lie was transverse and the fetal elbow was protruding through the cervix. She was in danger of a having a ruptured uterus, the fetus was in danger of dying. The situation was desperate and there was little time to act. On religious grounds she refused to have the operation and her husband supported the decision. She was undoubtedly competent to make the decision.

The obstetricians applied to the court for a declaration that to do the operation without the woman's consent would not be unlawful. The decision made by the Family Division of the High Court was made very rapidly. The application went to the Court at 1.30pm and at 2.18pm the judge, Sir Stephen Brown, declared that it would, under the circumstances, be lawful to carry out the caesarean section. Mrs S was unrepresented at the hearing.

Being only a High Court decision, this case is not binding on subsequent decisions. There was however, as with the case in America, an outcry following this decision, not the least from lawyers who all challenged it. A barrister, Barbara Hewson, writing in the *The Law Society Gazette* suggested that the case was discriminatory. She said

> 'The argument that pregnant women should forfeit their rights to bodily integrity is discriminatory. No competent man would be forced to undergo bodily invasion for his own or another's benefit. Nor would a parent have to undergo surgery for a born child ... Court-ordered Caesareans infringe basic rights to bodily integrity, a fair trial and equal treatment. They allow doctors to engage in indefensible practices in the name of defensive medicine, and judges to invade

women's personal and ethical decisions on health-care, when mani-
festly ill-equipped to do so . . . Pregnant women should not be put off
medical care for fear of forced surgery.' [1]

It would be surprising, given the legal misgivings, if this decision were
to be repeated, but the outcome of any future application to the courts
cannot be wholly predicted. It is an issue upon which midwives should
act if any woman in the future is denied the right to decide against
having medical treatment however extreme the circumstances might
be.

## OBTAINING CONSENT IN MIDWIFERY PRACTICE

Most of the cases discussed in the previous section were based upon
doctor's care but all the principles apply to midwifery practice. Midwives
make autonomous decisions about when or whether to give certain
drugs, whether to perform an episiotomy and suture the perineum, in
some places whether to augment labour, even whether to give a baby a
formula feed. Consent for these 'treatments' as well as for all other
clinical activity is necessary.

She is also a member of a team which looks after the woman during
pregnancy as well as labour and so has the opportunity to give the
woman information on which she can base her consent to treatment.
This can be very important when subsequently managing labour. Take
the following example:

### Case study: urgent episiotomy

Gill is helping Debbie during the second stage of labour. Progress is fairly
good but there is some delay as the head descends onto the perineum. Gill
has some concern about the condition of the fetus and decides to do an
episiotomy. She tells Debbie what she is going to do and, because of the
need to act quickly, immediately performs the episiotomy.

This is of course a very common situation and requires the practitioner
to act without delay. Usually no subsequent problems arise. From a
consensual point of view it is no different from the case study of Angela
and Carol and the emergency caesarean section, except that in this
situation there is no doubt about Debbie's competence to consent.

Almost a year later, Gill was very upset when she was called to see her
manager and supervisor of midwives. She was told that they have
received a complaint from a solicitor acting for Debbie. She is still
having considerable pain from the episiotomy scar and this is severely
affecting sexual intercourse. She remembers that Gill told her that she
was going to 'cut her to open her up a bit more because her baby was

tired'. She claims that she had no time to agree or otherwise, she knew nothing about how the operation would be done and no idea about any adverse effects there might be. She claims that Gill had been negligent in giving information to her.

Gill is asked to make a statement. The delivery was routine and Gill cannot remember any of the detailed facts of her care. She is given the case notes to help her and she contacts her professional organization which arranges for her to have help.

The reference in the kardex to the episiotomy reads,

'Episiotomy performed for fetal distress'.

Later it says,

'Episiotomy sutured with Dexon'

and, in the postnatal notes,

'Perineum painful. Some suture material removed'.

There is no record of any discussions that may have taken place on the use and effects of episiotomy and no record that consent was obtained.

Debbie was a primigravida. Gill's representative suggested that she might have attended antenatal classes so she may have had a discussion on episiotomy during pregnancy. They contacted the community midwife but, although she could confirm that Debbie came to the classes, she could not confirm that she had specifically been at the class where episiotomy was discussed. The community midwife did say that she did not usually talk too much about subsequent dyspareunia as it might make women anxious.

### Potential Pitfalls

There are a number of points to make about this situation.

(1) If Debbie's version of the events is true, it is possible she did not give consent to the episiotomy. Unless she was given the time to agree it is difficult to see how she could have either implied her consent or expressly withheld consent at the time just before delivery.

(2) She could therefore claim, using the civil action of trespass to the person. She has not done so, however, because there are few successful cases and her solicitor probably would have advised her against it.

(3) Her claim that there was negligence in not giving her sufficient information is more likely to succeed.

(4) It is not surprising that the two midwives, Gill and the community

midwife, have some difficulty in recalling important facts; but the midwifery notes are not very helpful.

(5) There is no record of the classes that Debbie attended or the topics that were covered, so the notes cannot corroborate the possible defence that Debbie had discussions antenatally.

(6) There is no record in the labour notes that consent was obtained to do the episiotomy. Consent can of course be given verbally, but a contemporaneous record should be made as verbal consent is more difficult to prove convincingly than written consent.

## Possible defences

The defence could use two arguments.

The community midwife could confirm that her classes always contain a discussion on the episiotomy and so if Debbie went to all the classes she would have been involved in that discussion. On the other hand, Debbie would probably not have been told about possible dyspareunia but, if it could be shown that a significant number of midwives would also not mention it, it is unlikely that negligence would be found in this respect.

Gill could ask for expert witnesses, other midwives, to show that a body of responsible professional opinion would also have done the episiotomy and, under the circumstances and given the need to act quickly, would have told Debbie about doing it in the same way – in effect using the principles of the *Bolam* test.

### Steps for prevention

All this could have been avoided if the midwifery service had thought carefully about giving advice as being a part of consent to treatment and not just to prepare women for labour and baby care.

Also if a record had been kept of the classes that Debbie had attended, with the topics that had been discussed, then it could have been shown that she had been given the information. On the other hand, had she missed the class on episiotomy, then Gill would have seen this in the notes when she admitted Debbie in labour and could have used the time she was looking after her to fill the gap, discussing the implications of possible procedures she might need to use.

The midwives should also consider using booklets to give information. Again, if they are to rely on giving written information on possible treatments, it is probably best if this is recorded. Even though there is a time limit of three years for Debbie to bring an action, three years is far too long to remember whether she was given an explanatory booklet which would have covered episiotomy.

## Homebirth – a special case

Although most women who have a homebirth do so with the full support of the professional team caring for them, there are circumstances when a woman chooses to have her baby at home against the professional advice of a midwife or doctor.

In essence this is a case of refusal of advised care and is one of the more common situations involving consent to treatment. The law does not expressly require a professional to give treatment when in her judgment it is unwise to do so. The midwife will not be obliged in law to attend a delivery at home if she has advised that it is ill-judged. If things go wrong during the birth the midwife would still be held liable and could be found to be negligent in her actions. It would, however, be much more difficult in such circumstances for the woman to prove causation (that the midwife's actions caused the damage) and, even if causation were proved, it would be open to the midwife to raise the woman's contributory negligence thus limiting the case against herself.

Although in law there would be no obligation to attend such a case, it is very likely that the UKCC would view failure to continue to give care as professional misconduct. It has, however, given useful guidance on what to do in these cases. It is given in A Midwife's Code of Practice, section 4.

This section is a prime example of risk management. It accepts there may be situations which can lead to difficulties and gives guidance and a framework of action to minimize any adverse outcome. It covers:

- the availability or otherwise of a medical practitioner,
- the midwife's continuing duty to the woman,
- the role of the supervisor, and
- the advisability of having pre-agreed local policies to enable the midwife to have appropriate support if she has to attend a woman at home where there are contra-indications to this.

## Getting consent during pregnancy

Although it is good practice to give information on which a woman can base her consent to treatment during pregnancy, can consent itself be obtained in anticipation of the treatments that may be necessary?

### Birth plans

Many maternity services now encourage the use of a birth plan which the woman completes giving her wishes for care. These plans can be relied upon as indicating her consent to the type of care she has asked for as long as she has had the opportunity to discuss all the options for care and understands the implications of her choices.

They should not be taken as the final consent to treatment. For example she may request not to have artificial rupture of membranes (ARM) in labour. This request should be honoured but time should be taken to inform her of the indications for doing an ARM. The onus for her having this information rests with the practitioner and not with the woman. The woman must also always have the opportunity to change her mind, and it is the responsibility of the midwife to keep her informed of any change in circumstances which may lead her to change her request. If therefore ARM is indicated, perhaps to attach a fetal scalp electrode, this should be discussed with her again and either her consent obtained, or her continued wish not to have it done reaffirmed.

It is very unwise to rely upon 'consent' given some time before the procedure is indicated. It should always be sought as near to the procedure as possible. Thus the birth plan should be seen only as an indicator of consent. It is also inappropriate to have a consent form signed as a 'blanket consent' for any possible treatment.

### The Department of Health Guide

The Department of Health issued a comprehensive guide to consent to treatment in 1990. This covers the general principles of consent, including a summary of the main legal background. It gives standard consent forms, including one for health professionals other than doctors and dentists.

There is a section on consent in maternity services. This states:

'(1) Principles of consent are the same in maternity services as in other areas of medicine. It is important that the proposed care is discussed with the woman, preferably in the early antenatal period, when any special wishes she expresses should be recorded in the notes, but of course the patient may change her mind about these issues at any stage, including during labour.

(2) Decisions may have to be taken swiftly at a time when the woman's ability to give consent is impaired, e.g. as a result of medication, including analgesics. If the safety of the woman or child is at stake the obstetrician should take any reasonable action that is necessary. If, in the judgment of the relevant health professional, the woman is temporarily unable to make a decision, it may be advisable for the position to be explained to her husband or partner, if available, but his consent (or withholding of consent) cannot legally over-ride the clinical judgment of the health professional, as guided by the previously expressed wishes of the patient herself.' [2]

For midwives it should be added that if treatment has to be carried out without the consent of the woman because her ability to consent is judged to be impaired, it would be wise to discuss this with the supervisor of midwives and make sure that there is a record of this discussion in the notes. Also it is probably wise to write a personal statement at the time, and keep this safe yourself.

# CONSENT TO TREATMENT – A RISK MANAGEMENT APPROACH

As with negligence it is advisable to introduce working practices to ensure as far as possible that informed consent will always be obtained or, where it cannot be, that proper action is taken in the interests of the woman and the health professionals. This is best done with agreement of the professional disciplines involved so that they all follow the same general principles and also understand the specific requirements for each separate profession.

A few simple questions, based upon the legal principles given earlier in this chapter, will help to formulate a policy for getting informed consent and avoiding any claims that it had not been obtained.

- Is express consent obtained for all invasive procedures?

- If the consent is obtained in writing, is the relevant standard form used?

- If the consent is given verbally, is it contemporaneously recorded in the notes?

- Does each woman receive information that will help her to make a decision about her consent to a treatment?

- Is there a record of her having this information, including the circumstances and the form in which it was given?

- Would a responsible body of professional midwifery opinion agree with the information that is given and the way in which consent is obtained?

- If consent is not possible because of the woman's lack of competence to give it, is this always recorded, with the reason why she was not able to give consent?

- If she is unable to give consent, is this discussed with her husband or partner, and is this discussion always recorded?

- Is failure to obtain consent discussed with the supervisor of midwives and is this discussion recorded?

- Are clinical notes systematically audited for evidence that informed consent to treatment is always obtained?

## SUMMARY

Adults of sound mind have the right to consent to or withhold consent for medical treatment. Treatment carried out without consent could be battery.

The health care professional has a duty to give a patient information on which to base a decision to have treatment or not. Failure to give the information that a reasonable body of professional opinion would give could be negligence.

Special circumstances exist for minors and those with mental impairment who may not be competent to give consent.

Despite *Re S* (1992), the right of the woman to consent to treatment or withhold it, even if not in the best interests of her unborn child, is usually paramount.

To avoid a claim that informed consent was not obtained maternity services should introduce policies that ensure information is given and consent obtained, and that both are recorded for all appropriate 'treatments'.

## FURTHER ACTION

- Obtain and read the Department of Health booklet, *A Guide to Consent to Treatment*.

- Discuss introducing unit/practice policies to ensure that informed consent to treatment is obtained and recorded.

- Set up an audit of midwifery notes to see whether informed consent is obtained and can be proved.

## REFERENCES

1. Hewson, B. *The Law Society Gazette*, **89**, (45) 9th December 1992.
2. Department of Health, *Health Circular: A Guide to Consent for Examination or Treatment*. HC (90)22. London. DoH, 1990.

# Chapter 7
# Holding Information

During the course of her work, the midwife has access to a wide range of information which is often confidential.

- She has the clinical information that she has obtained herself.
- She has clinical information from other professionals, either reported to her verbally or written in the clinical notes.
- She finds out about the families of women she is looking after.
- She has information about her colleagues.
- She has information about her employer – working practices, future plans, perhaps financial information.

This chapter will look at the legal and ethical principles that should guide the midwife about the appropriate use and storage of this information. As with other areas of practice, the legal requirements can be found in common law, in statute and in the requirements of the UKCC.

## CONFIDENTIALITY

The overriding principle relating to clinical information is that it is confidential. If it is passed on without the permission of the person who has given it she could claim that the information was negligently communicated.

## Exceptions to the rule

This general rule of confidentiality does have exceptions. Information can be given to others in the following circumstances.

(1) If the person giving the information consents to the disclosure of information.

(2) On a need-to-know basis. In the health care context the passing of

information to other health care workers on a need-to-know basis would fall into this category. Obviously it is in the best interests of a patient that all those professionals involved in the care share information in order to provide continuity of treatment.

(3) In the public interest. For example, if a midwife found that one of her clients or a member of her family has committed a serious crime she may pass the information on if appropriate. This may not be simple because if the misdemeanour is not serious its disclosure may be found to have broken confidentiality. If the midwife has been made aware of information which might have to be disclosed in the public interest she should discuss it with her supervisor of midwives. If the supervisor is also unclear of what to do, she should refer it to her managers and ask if the employer's lawyers could give legal advice. Seeking advice about a matter within the employing authority would not be construed a breach of confidentiality.

(4) Because there is a statutory duty to disclose the information. An example of this is the requirement to notify infectious diseases. There is a specific list of diseases which fall into this category, which includes ophthalmia neonatorum, rubella and food poisoning. This latter category would include listeriosis if diagnosed in pregnancy.

(5) Because there is a court order to disclose information. The Supreme Court Act 1981 requires that medical records relating to litigation should be released to the plaintiff's lawyers prior to a court hearing.

### The Supreme Court Act and medical records

The last category enumerated above includes medical and midwifery notes, and other relevant material such as X-rays, test results, CTG recordings, reports and letters that have been generated during the course of treatment. Although the Act lays down a process by which the documents will be released on a court order, it is becoming more usual for the health authority or Trust to release the information automatically on application.

Pre-trial disclosure of the reports of expert and non-expert witnesses is also required by the Act. The records and reports are not released directly to the plaintiff.

The only documents which may be withheld are the reports into a medical mishap which are prepared afterwards and specifically to counter a possible legal claim. This would not apply if they were made for a purpose other than potential litigation.

## Requirements of the UKCC

A breach of confidentiality could also lead to a charge of professional misconduct and if proved, the midwife's name could be removed from the Register.

Paragraph 10 of the Code of Professional Conduct of the UKCC states:

> 'As a registered nurse, midwife or health visitor, you are personally accountable for your practice and, in the exercise of your professional accountability, must ... protect all confidential information concerning patients and clients obtained in the course of professional practice and make disclosures only with consent, where required by the order of a court or where you can justify disclosure in the wider public interest.' [1]

This is further elaborated in a separate guidance document on confidentiality [2] which confirms that patients or clients have the right to expect confidentiality and that the death of a patient/client does not absolve the practitioner from this obligation.

# Confidentiality – some ethical dilemmas

## In someone else's best interests?

There may be times when confidentiality towards a patient may result in an increased risk to someone else and the professional may be faced with a difficult ethical dilemma. Consider the following situation:

> Catherine, an independent midwife, has been approached by Margaret who is pregnant and wants non-NHS care. However, a week after booking, she rings Catherine up an asks to see her urgently. When Catherine arrives at her house, Margaret is alone and very upset. She explains that she has just been to her general practitioner. Some time ago she had a short affair with a man and subsequently found out that he might be HIV positive. She decided to be tested and had just heard that she also is HIV positive. She wants a termination of pregnancy and the general practitioner is willing to arrange this. However, she does not want her husband to know about her sero-positive state or about the termination. She asks Catherine, therefore, not to say anything to her husband. She asks Catherine to send her a bill for any professional services she has given so far, and not to call again. Margaret and her husband have one three-year old daughter who appears to be very healthy.

This situation raises some very difficult dilemmas for the general practitioner and the midwife. Positive HIV status is not a communicable disease so there is no statutory obligation to disclose it.

For the general practitioner there is an additional dilemma. Margaret's husband is also one of his patients and he therefore has a duty of care towards him. Of course the way to deal with this situation is to discuss the implications of her decision with Margaret and the effect that not telling her husband might have. He may already be infected but if not steps should be taken to protect him. She should understand the effect there may be to her daughter who may lose both parents.

In this situation the midwife should discuss what she has been told with Margaret's general practitioner. He will probably arrange to counsel her carefully.

If a midwife ever found herself in a situation like this, she should certainly discuss whether to disclose the information to Margaret's husband with her supervisor of midwives. It is such a difficult professional decision to make she and the supervisor may consider asking for guidance from the UKCC.

The general practitioner would be advised to approach the General Medical Council for similar help if he is unsure what to do.

### Confidentiality in criminal cases

The following case study illustrates a situation that occasionally confronts midwives.

> Penny is Vanessa's midwife. She has seen Vanessa in the antenatal clinic because this has been her wish. However, Vanessa has not attended for two of her appointments so Penny calls at her flat. Vanessa somewhat reluctantly lets Penny into the flat and Penny is surprised to see that the living room is full of boxes of hi-fi equipment. Vanessa breaks down and tells Penny that the equipment is stolen and that her husband has been involved for some time in receiving stolen goods. Penny reports this confidentially to her supervisor and they decide that it would not be in Vanessa's interests to report it. They do nothing. A few weeks later, Penny is visited at home by two policemen who ask if she will be a police witness to testify against Vanessa's husband. Penny says she must discuss this with her manager and asks them to contact her again when she has sought advice. The police tell her that they will issue a subpoena to require her to attend court if she does not agree to help.

Penny's first reaction was correct. A midwife finding herself in this situation should seek the immediate guidance of both her supervisor and her employing authority.

Giving confidential information gained in the course of professional attendance could be professional misconduct. It could also lead to a claim against the employing authority who could be vicariously liable for negligent disclosure of information.

From a personal point of view, Penny has built up a good professional relationship with Vanessa which she does not want to break. On the other hand, she knows she cannot ignore a subpoena if it is served on her as she would be found in contempt of court.

Because of this, Penny will have to go to court if the police require it. She should discuss very carefully with her managers the information she is likely to be asked. Of course in this case she is unlikely to be asked to give clinical information, rather what she saw in the flat during her visit. Penny should ask to talk to her employers' lawyers to get legal advice about what she might disclose and what information she should keep confidential.

Even during the trial, if Penny is asked to give information that she feels unhappy about, she can seek direction from the judge. He will give guidance about whether she should give or withhold information.

# OWNERSHIP AND STORAGE OF MIDWIFERY RECORDS

## Who the records belong to

Ownership of records made by a health care professional will depend upon whether the person is self-employed or an employee. The usual rule is that a record belongs to the person who has written it. However, if the practitioner is an employee then ownership rests with the generator of the document and therefore with the employer. Thus the notes a midwife makes in the course of her work which use the standard clinical form belong to her employer. But if she makes a personal record of any of the care she gives, this would belong to her. Clinical notes do not belong the patient or client, although as seen below she may hold them during her pregnancy.

Rule 42 of the Midwives Rules states:

'A midwife must not destroy or arrange for the destruction of official records which have been made whilst she is in professional atten- dance upon a case (for the purpose of the rule called "official records"). If she finds it impossible or inconvenient to preserve her official records safely she must transfer them to the local supervising authority or to her employing authority and details of the transfer must be duly recorded by each party to the transfer.'

The midwife who is employed must pass her records to the LSA immediately before retirement whilst the self-employed midwife may do so.

The Code of Practice requires that the form of record used by the self-employed midwife must be approved by the LSA.

## Department of Health guidelines

One of the important reasons to keep records is in case of future liti- gation. Although the Limitation Act 1980 generally excludes an action after three years, this is different in maternity care. The Department of Health issued a guidance document, *Preservation of Records*, in 1989. This requires that.

> 'obstetric records must be retained for 25 years; or 8 years after the death of child (but not mother) if sooner.'

It also states:

> 'Obstetric claims: these are perhaps the most important exception both to the Department's guidance on retention of records, and to the general three-year time limit. Time does not run against a minor litigant, for the purposes of the Act, until he or she reaches the age of 18 years. A Writ can therefore be issued just before the plaintiff's 21st birthday . . . It is for this reason that the Department specifies a period of retention of 25 years for obstetric records. Claims concerning alleged birth injury dating back to the 1970s (and even earlier) are relatively common and invariably quite expensive. These claims are often difficult to investigate, even with the aid of comprehensive records including such important items as the fetal heart trace (where these exist).' [3]

## Form of storage

There is no legal requirement that controls the form in which medical records should be stored and electronic storage and microfiche may be used more in the future.

Increasingly, now, records are being initially generated using computer systems such as the well established St Mary's computerized records (the St Mary's Maternity Information System – SMMIS). The same legal principles apply. They should be secure and maintain confidentiality.

This can usually be achieved using password entry to restrict the number of people who can have access to the data. It must be possible to identify the timing of all entries and the identity of the person putting data into the notes as well as the person who was responsible for the clinical activity. At present most systems also generate a printout which can be stored as a manual record. The UKCC has considered computerized records in its publication *Standards for Records and Record Keeping* [4]. It advises that local protocols

> 'must include means of authenticating an entry in the absence of a written signature and must indicate clearly the identity of the originator of that entry.'

# Women-held Records

There are sound clinical reasons why women should have access to their maternity record. Holding their own notes will also go a long way to satisfy recent legal requirements regarding patients' access to health care information.

Women are increasingly holding their own maternity notes, rather than the short summary they used to have in the form of the now obsolete 'co-operation card'. These notes are used by all the professionals that give her care. If care is given in the NHS, these notes belong to the employer and not to any one professional group. An employer can therefore make the decision on jointly used notes although this is always done with the agreement of all concerned.

The recent NHS Management Executive circular on *Changing Childbirth* has reiterated that all women should hold their own notes within five years. This should not create any legal problems. Many studies of the system show that fewer notes are lost by women than by the medical records departments.

It will not expose the negligent practitioner any more than at present because if a writ is served the plaintiff's lawyers are in any event given full copies of the notes. In fact it could improve matters as the professional is likely to take more care in completing notes if she knows that the woman will see what is written.

Looking to the future, there are already local studies on the possibility of computerized notes held by women on a SMART card. They have access to a computer terminal in the antenatal clinic and are shown how to read the information held on the card.

# THE PATIENT'S STATUTORY RIGHTS

## The Data Protection Act 1984

The Data Protection Act 1984 came into force in 1987. It gave people the right to know what is held about them on computer. The Act is general and not specifically for medical information but it applies equally to health related data.

The main provisions of the Act are that:

- Anyone who holds information on computer about individuals must register and not to do so is a criminal offence.

- The data can only be held if it conforms to certain statutory principles (given below).

- Individuals about whom data is held have the right to know what that data is.

- A Data Protection Tribunal hears appeals from people who feel that the data principles have been contravened.

### Principles of good practice

The principles are contained in Schedule 1 of the Act. There are eight of them.

(1) The data should be obtained and processed fairly and lawfully.

(2) The data should be held only for specified and lawful purposes.

(3) The data should not be disclosed other than for purposes given at registration.

(4) The data held should be adequate for the purpose for which it is held and should not be excessive.

(5) The data should be accurate.

(6) The data should be kept for no longer than is necessary.

(7) An individual shall be entitled:
   (a) to be informed whether data is held about him,
   (b) to have access to that data, and
   (c) to have any inaccurate data corrected.

(8) Appropriate security measures should be adopted to prevent unauthorised access, disclosure or loss of personal data held.

### Exceptions under the Act

The Act allows for the holding of personal data for historic, statistical or research purposes providing it is not used in such a way as to cause damage or distress and that it was not obtained unfairly. For these purposes the information may be held indefinitely.

An exemption to the provisions of the Act was introduced in 1987 with the Data Protection (Subject Access Modification) (Health) Order. This restricted access to health information which might cause serious harm to physical or mental health, or to that of another individual, or where it might reveal the identity of another person.

## The Access to Health Records Act 1990

The passing of the Data Protection Act 1984 created an anomaly. Whilst people whose medical records were held on computer could have access to them, freedom of access to manually held records was not a statutory right.

To correct this the Access to Health Records Act 1990 was passed. It came into force in November 1991. This Act builds upon the 1984 Act and brings together all the statutory requirements for access to the medical record.

The purpose of the Act is to give a person or his authorized representative the right to apply to see their health record, or any part of it, in whatever form the record is held. It can be the record made by any of the health professionals who are listed in the Act, which includes registered nurses, midwives and health visitors, but it only applies to records made after November 1991. Access to records made earlier will only be permitted if it is required to clarify the meaning of a record made after November 1991.

## Applications

When an application is made to see the medical record, subject to statutory exemption the record or relevant part record should be made available. If the record was made within 40 days of the application, it should be made available within 21 days; if the record was made some time ago, it should be made available within 40 days. The patient may ask for a copy to be made of the notes.

A fee may be charged, not exceeding that laid down in the Data Protection Act 1984, for releasing records made more than 40 days ago, and a charge can be made to cover the cost of making a copy.

## Exclusions

The Act allows for the same exclusions that were originally described under the Data Protection Order.

Records can be withheld if the applicant is a child and it is thought that he would not understand the nature of the application, and if it is thought that the patient has not consented to the application.

Partial exemption is granted if, in the opinion of the holder of the record, the information may cause serious harm or if it identifies a third party.

## Consultation

The Act imposes a duty upon a health service body to consult with the relevant health professional if an application to have access to the medical record has been made. This is usually the doctor in charge of the case, but may be

'a health professional who has the necessary experience and qualifications to advise the body on the matter in question.'

In the circumstances where a midwife is the lead professional in a woman's care, or where the part of the record has been generated by a midwife, it is likely that the midwife will be the professional consulted by the health service body.

### Responsibilities of the self-employed midwife

This Act is not confined to health service activity, and application to see the midwifery records of a self-employed midwife can be made under the Act. She would be advised to discuss the application with her supervisor of midwives particularly if she believes that for some reason part or all of the record should be withheld. Any decision to withhold information should be recorded in a statement giving the reasons for doing so.

### Corrections and intelligibility

There are two other important provisions of the Act.

Where the person considers the health record to be inaccurate he may apply for it to be corrected. If the holder of the record agrees that it is inaccurate, the Act allows for the record to be corrected. If the holder disagrees, she should make a note in the record about the areas of disagreement.

In both these circumstances, the midwife may be required to alter her clinical record. She should consult with the supervisor of midwives about this and it would be wise to keep a personal statement about the reasons for the change to her clinical notes. She should ask the supervisor to witness the change in the notes so that, if they are returned to later, there is a full explanation for the altered record.

The second provision in the Act is that the notes must be made available in a form that will be intelligible to the patient. If they are not, the professional may be asked to re-write them or write explanatory notes so that they can be understood. This would particularly apply to the use of abbreviations but may apply if the handwriting is poor. Rather than wait until a request is received to re-write the notes clearly, it is advisable to write the notes clearly and comprehensibly in the first place.

### Time limits

Receiving an application to give access to clinical notes can be complicated yet the Act imposes a strict time deadline on the process. Figure 7.1 gives a flowchart which, if followed, will ensure that none of the steps are omitted.

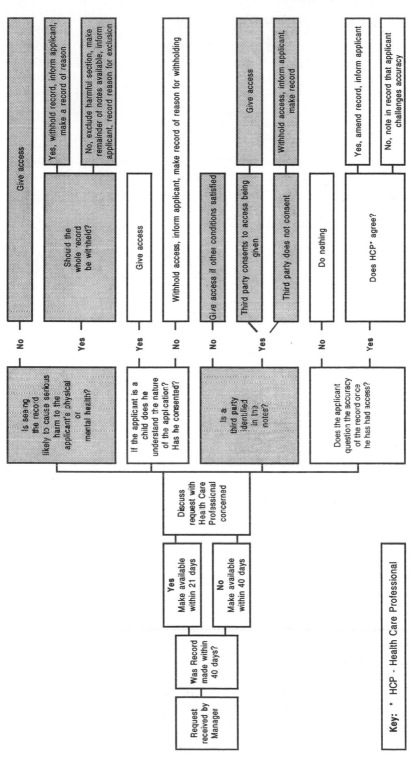

**Fig. 7.1** Flowchart for responding to a request for information from medical notes.

## RECORD KEEPING IN PRACTICE

The clinical record by the health professional, made contemporaneously with the care or treatment given, is one of the most effective ways of protecting the practitioner and her employer from the vagaries of the law. There is no common law requirement to keep records, but the Midwives Rules impose a duty upon the practising midwife to

'keep as contemporaneously as is reasonable detailed records of observations, care given and medicine or other forms of pain relief administered by her to all mothers and babies.'

Failure to meet this requirement could lead to a charge of professional misconduct.

The UKCC booklet, *Standards for Records and Record Keeping*, [4] gives five problems associated with inadequate record keeping which it says neglects clients' interests through

(1) impairing continuity of care;
(2) introducing discontinuity of communication between staff;
(3) creating the risk of medication or other treatment being duplicated or omitted;
(4) failing to focus attention on early signs of deviation from the norm; and
(5) failing to place on record significant observations and conclusions.

In addition to these points, the clinical record is one of the most important ways that the midwife can prove what care she gave, especially if some time has elapsed since the events.

Well made records should:

- be contemporaneous,
- be legible,
- have clarity of meaning,
- show the timing and sequence of events accurately, and
- have a distinguishable signature.

Any deletions should be a single line so that the original wording can be seen. Any alteration should have the time, date and signature and, if necessary, an explanation for the alteration.

If some recordings of care are kept as separate data items (for example, the partogram and a CTG trace) the information in them must not conflict; this is particularly the case with the timing of events on each of the recordings.

Particular care should be taken with the CTG. Any automatic timing that shows on the trace should be checked at the beginning of the trace and regularly throughout the labour. When significant treatments are carried out, such as a vaginal examination, these should also be indicated and if there is a possible abnormality on the trace this should be noted including the action that is taken.

Midwifery records should also show the decisions that are made regarding clinical management and not just the treatments and observations that are carried out. Clinical decisions may range between deciding to do nothing but be extra vigilant, to deciding to alter the management or to call for medical aid.

When notes are being scrutinized so that a statement can be written or for the purposes of a potential legal case, difficulties in their interpretation are commonly caused because:

- two different records have conflicting information;

- it is difficult to determine the actual sequence of events during the clinical management;

- there are apparent gaps in the observations;

- adverse observations may be recorded or there is an indication that the management of a case has changed, but there is no record of the clinical decision that the midwife has made;

- it is not possible to ascertain from the signatures who carried out the care or the observations; or

- the use of non-standard abbreviations leads to a lack of clarity.

## The future maternity record

Now that *Changing Childbirth* has set a target that all women should carry their maternity notes, consideration should be given to the use of a single record contributed to by all the professional groups giving care. The format of such notes must be agreed between the different groups so that their varying needs to record information particular to their sphere of practice are met.

Apart from the advantage to the woman of having access to one set of cohesive notes, another advantage is that the whole picture of the clinical management is much clearer. Whether a midwife carries out a particular procedure before or after a doctor does something is immediately apparent if both practitioners are using the same notes and recording everything in time sequence. Time intervals can be better assessed. In many cases there is some doubt about the time between a midwife calling for medical aid and the doctor arriving. Again the confusion is often made worse because the midwife makes her recording in one set of notes and the doctor uses another set.

There are circumstances when women receive some care in one NHS Trust and then transfer to another Trust. This may be for clinical reasons but also may be the result of the woman's preference for care elsewhere. With a much more flexible service midwives may also work across different maternity service boundaries as they increasingly meet women's needs for continuity of carer.

There may now be a strong argument for the development of a national standard maternity record which will be used by all clinical staff wherever the woman receives her care. Coupled with an increasing awareness of the importance of accurate record keeping, a standardized approach to the format of records, especially if agreed by the various professional bodies representing the professions involved, may act as a major risk management tool as well as aiding more continuity of clinical care.

# AUDIT, RESEARCH AND CONFIDENTIAL ENQUIRY

Audit, research and confidential enquiry are three techniques for the development of clinical knowledge and the improvement and maintenance of standards. All three however depend upon the use of clinical information which may have been obtained confidentially. Midwives are increasingly involved in all three activities so should have a clear understanding of how the duty of care regarding this information can be met.

## Audit

Audit should rarely present problems. It is usually a process of measuring care given or outcomes achieved, such as the episiotomy rate, the breast feeding rate or the number of women attending antenatal classes. The collection of this information does not involve information that might have been derived confidentially from a woman or her family, but all audit activity should be carefully assessed to ensure that confidential information is not made known inadvertently.

Audit of patient satisfaction as an outcome may seek to obtain confidential information in the questionnaire. For example, a midwifery practice may want to audit the outcome of perineal care and may want to know how many women are still experiencing pain after a specified period of time. This would be highly sensitive and confidential information. The midwives could consider a number of approaches.

They may make the questionnaire completely confidential so that it is returned anonymously. The advantage of this approach is the anonymity of the returns. This may be a reassurance to the women asked to complete the form and may therefore result in a higher return rate. The disadvantage is that individual adverse reports cannot be referred back to the original case management to find out if there were factors which may have contributed to the poor outcome.

They may identify the questionnaire with an anonymized code which could be used to trace the reply back to the specific case notes. If this approach is used, great care in the data processing must be adopted so that those midwives who have the information subsequently sent back to them will only be those who have a right to it on a need-to-know basis.

# Research

If an audit activity is likely to generate data based on information gained confidentially, it is probably safer to treat it as potential research and use the rigorous approach that research based on clinical information demands.

Much research in medicine and midwifery, whether large multi-centre trials or local research, depends upon the processing of confidential clinical information. Safeguards must be built into all research projects to protect the patients from inadvertent disclosure of information and to protect the professional from accusations of negligent disclosure.

All the stages of a research project should be carefully designed so that the only information to be collected and processed is that which is necessary to the project. The stages are:

- piloting the project,
- data collection,
- data analysis,
- the research report.

Any ensuing publication must be designed to protect the information that has been made available to the project. To make certain that this is the case, research projects should be submitted to a multi-disciplinary ethical committee for its adjudication on whether the data subject's rights are preserved. Projects when under way should not deviate from the agreed protocols. If part way through the research there needs to be change in an agreed protocol, this should be referred back to the committee for further approval.

The other protection for the researchers who will be handling clinical information is to obtain the informed consent of all the people who enrol into the project. The information upon the basis of which the patient's consent will be given should include:

- a summary of the research objectives;
- the information that is to be collected;

- how it will be collected and analysed; who will have access to the information; and
- how it will eventually be reported.

All potential research subjects should have the opportunity to refuse involvement so that their agreement to participate is actively sought rather than passively obtained.

## Confidential enquiry

The confidential enquiry is a unique form of audit where individual case notes are subjected to professional scrutiny to identify sub-standard care. Maternity services have two national confidential enquiries, the long established Enquiry into Maternal Mortality and the recently introduced Confidential Enquiry into Stillbirths and Deaths in Infancy (CESDI). Midwives have been involved in all levels of CESDI from its inception and in 1994 it was announced that midwives would also be included in the assessment stages of the Maternal Mortality Survey. There is a third national confidential enquiry, which is unlikely to involve maternity cases but looks at peri-operative death, the Confidential Enquiry into Peri-operative Death.

These enquiries are administered and supported by the Department of Health but are reliant upon regional level clinical assessment as well as a national overview. Confidentiality is maintained

- by anonymizing the clinical notes,
- discussion of clinical management at closed meetings,
- by not photocopying or posting data, and
- by altering the information in the final published report so that it cannot be traced back to the actual events.

The processes are constantly reviewed by the Department to ensure that they continue to remain anonymous.

Midwives involved in either the death of a woman or a baby may be required to complete forms giving detailed information about the case so that it can be assessed by the confidential enquiry process. They should be assured that this information will be treated confidentially and at the local district level will be anonymized to protect confidentiality. The midwife would not be at risk of failing in her duty of care to her clients if she carefully follows the instructions she is given when compiling information for these studies.

## SUMMARY

The midwife receives a large volume of information in the course of her work.

She has a duty of care to keep confidential information confidential and, if she does not, could be found to be negligent or guilty of professional misconduct

The Access to Health Records Act 1990 gives patients the right to see their medical notes, whether held on computer or manually, although information can be withheld if it is anticipated that it may cause physical or mental harm or may identify a third party.

Accurate record keeping is not only imperative to maintaining high standards of clinical care, it is required by the Midwives Rules and is a valuable aid to proving the clinical care that was given when a legal claim is made.

Audit, research and confidential enquiry need particular care to preserve confidentiality of information.

## FURTHER ACTION

- Find out whether there is a local procedure for giving access to medical records, whether there is a designated manager who deals with it in your employing authority and how many requests there have been.

- Hold a meeting in your unit/practice to audit a sample of the notes to ask whether:

    - all the entries are clear and signed,
    - the time sequence of care given is clear and
    - the clinical decision making is clear.

- If women do not hold their notes at the moment, suggest that the midwives meet to discuss how to introduce it.

- Find out about membership of the local ethical committee and whether midwives as well as obstetricians sit on it when maternity research is considered.

## REFERENCES

1. United Kingdom Central Council for Nursing, Midwifery and Health Visiting. *Code of Professional Conduct for the Nurse, Midwife and Health Visitor*, London, UKCC, 1992.
2. United Kingdom Central Council for Nursing, Midwifery and Health Visiting. *Confidentiality: An Elaboration of Clause 9 of the Second Edition of the UKCC's Code of Professional Conduct for the Nurse. Midwife and Health Visitor.* London, UKCC 1987.
3. Department of Health. *Health Circular: Preservation of Records.* HC (89) 20, London, DoH, 1989.
4. United Kingdom Central Council for Nursing, Midwifery and Health Visiting. *Standards for Records and Record Keeping.* London, UKCC, 1993.

# Chapter 8
# Statutory Rights in Pregnancy

A little more than half the current workforce in the UK are now women. Patterns of work and family life have changed considerably in the past 20 years so that it is more usual for a woman to take maternity leave and then return to paid employment. Women have certain statutory rights to leave and benefits to enable them to have time off with an income during part of their pregnancy and after delivery. The benefit system is complicated and can be confusing so women often rely upon their midwife to explain their statutory rights.

There have been recent changes to the statutes which apply to maternity benefits which came into force on 16 October 1994. The following sections summarize the woman's entitlements. The Benefits Agency, an executive agency of the Department of Social Security, produces two booklets, *Which Benefit* and *Babies and Benefits* which give greater detail about maternity entitlements.

## MATERNITY ENTITLEMENTS

### Maternity leave

The Trade Union Reform and Employment Rights Act 1993 introduced changes to the statutory maternity leave by extending the right to have 14 weeks maternity leave to all women, regardless of their length of work, the hours of work or the size of their employer. This is a considerable improvement on the previous situation when women had to have worked for at least 16 hours a week for two years or over to qualify for the right to maternity leave.

The Act however still does not cover the woman who is self-employed. It also perpetuates a 'two-tier' system of right to maternity leave. The woman who has worked for two years full-time (over 16 hours per week) for her employer, or five years part-time (8 to 16 hours per week) still retains the additional right to 40 weeks leave, 11 weeks to be taken before the expected week of delivery and 29 weeks after the birth.

The following sections describe the main provisions of the current statutory position.

### Fourteen weeks leave

**Who benefits:** All women who are employed, regardless of the number of hours worked or length of service.

**Who is excluded:** Women who are self-employed.

**How do they obtain the leave:** The woman must write to her employer 21 days before she intends to take her leave giving details of when the baby is due and when she intends to take the leave. She should submit Form MAT B1 if her employer requires it. This is obtained from her doctor or midwife on or after the twenty eighth week of pregnancy. If she is admitted to hospital before she has given the required notice she should do so as soon as possible.

**When does the leave start:** She may start her leave eleven weeks before her baby is due but can stop work at any time after this. If however, she has a pregnancy related absence in the last six weeks of the pregnancy, even if of short duration, she may be required to continue her maternity leave whether she wishes to or not.

**Employment rights when on leave:** The woman's contractual rights continue whilst on leave (for example holiday entitlement) although her pay level will alter.

**Going back to work:** The woman has to give 14 days notice of return to work if she wishes to return early but not if she takes the whole leave entitlement. She has the right only to return back to the job she had before.

**Extension of the leave:** If the baby is born late it may be possible to extend the leave for up to two weeks. If at the end of the 14 weeks the woman is not well, the maternity leave will be converted to sick leave and she should be able to have statutory sick pay.

### Forty weeks leave

**Who benefits:** Women who have worked for the same employer for at least two years for 16 hours per week or over, or for five years between 8 and 16 hours per week. They must have completed this qualifying period of work by the twelfth week of the pregnancy.

**Who is excluded:** Women who are self-employed and women who have not worked for a the full qualifying period.

**How do they obtain the leave:** The woman must write to her employer at least 21 days before she intends to take the leave informing him

- that she will be taking leave,
- the expected date of the birth, and
- that she intends to return to work.

She may be required to submit Form MAT B1. As with the shorter leave entitlement, if she is unable to give 21 days notice because of intervening sickness, she should do so as soon as possible.

**When does the leave start:** These provisions are the same as for the shorter leave entitlement.

**Going back to work:** If the employer asks in writing whether the woman is intending to return, she must reply within 14 days confirming her intention to return. She must then, within 21 days of intended return, give notice of her intention to do so.

**Extension of the leave:** This can only be done if the woman is sick at the end of the leave and the extension will only be for up to four weeks. An application for extension must be accompanied by a medical certificate. The employer may also extend the leave by up to four weeks but must explain why in writing. An interruption to work, for example because of a strike, can legitimately delay a return to work.

## Maternity pay and allowances

The European Pregnant Workers Directive was adopted in October 1992 and the European states were required to implement its provisions by October 1994. The Directive laid down minimum levels of maternity pay that should be available throughout the European Union. These changes apply to all women whose expected date of delivery was on or after 16 October 1994.

As with the changes in the leave arrangements, there are improvements with the new statutory maternity pay; instead of the previous qualifying period of two years in work, this has now been reduced to 26 weeks. But again there are women who are still excluded from the benefit.

### Statutory Maternity Pay (SMP)

This is a weekly payment made to working women who are employed during pregnancy.

**Who can get SMP:** Women who have worked for the same employer for 26 weeks or more by the end of the fifteenth week before the expected date of delivery (EDD) and are still in employment. They must earn on average £57 per week or more. Women who have a stillbirth from the sixteenth week before the EDD can also receive SMP.

**How long does it last:** SMP is paid for up to 18 weeks and the woman can choose when this should start. It is not payable before the eleventh week prior to the EDD. This is an improvement from the previous situation when the woman received pay only up to six weeks after delivery regardless of when she finished work. The only exception to the woman's right to choose when to receive SMP is if she has a pregnancy related illness within the last six weeks of her pregnancy. She will then not be able to get statutory sick pay but will automatically receive SMP.

**How much will she get:** The woman will receive 90% of her average salary for the first six weeks of her leave and after that a basic rate (in 1994) of £52.50 per week for up to 12 weeks. The employer is expected to pay this and then get a full reimbursement of the payment from government funds.

**How will SMP be paid:** The woman must inform her employer 21 days before she intends to stop work and ask that SMP be paid. She must also send in Form MAT B1. It will attract any tax and national insurance contributions that will be due.

### Maternity Allowance

This is a weekly allowance for women who are in work before or during pregnancy but do not qualify for maternity pay.

**Who can get Maternity Allowance:** Self-employed women and those who changed jobs or gave up work during pregnancy.

**How much is it:** Two levels of allowance are available, £44.57 per week (in 1994) for the self-employed and recently unemployed; £52.50 for those who are employed in the fifteenth week prior to the EDD.

**How is it obtained:** The woman must complete Form MA1 and send it with Form MAT B1 to her Social Security office after the twenty sixth week of her pregnancy.

## Employment rights and benefits

### Employment rights

The Trade Union Reform and Employment Rights Act 1993 has changed the position regarding the woman's right not to be dismissed for pregnancy related reasons. Again the two or five year qualifying period has been abolished and all women will enjoy protection from dismissal for pregnancy reasons.

This protection has also been strengthened. The old legislation allowed an employer successfully to defend himself from a charge of unfair dismissal if he could prove that pregnancy or sickness related to pregnancy incapacitated the woman so that she could not work. This has been abolished. Importantly, however, a woman who loses her job in pregnancy and wishes to claim unfair dismissal must apply within three months of dismissal.

The 1993 Act also introduced a new health and safely protection for the pregnant woman and the woman who is breast feeding her baby. If the work conditions are deemed unsafe for the woman she should be offered alternative, safe employment and if this is not available she should be suspended on full pay. The employer will be expected to carry out health and safety checks to ensure that the working environment is safe for the pregnant woman.

A long standing right for pregnant women, first introduced in 1978, is the right to paid time off for antenatal care. Antenatal classes are also included for this purpose. The woman's employer may require her to obtain a certificate of attendance from the midwife or doctor and that may include confirmation that the woman will be attending classes. If a woman is denied this time off or pay while she is away from work she may apply to an industrial tribunal, but must do so within three months.

### Maternity benefits: problems and controversies

Although the benefits for pregnant women have been improved over the years there are still some significant criticisms of the system. These can be summarized as:

- The incompleteness of coverage.
- Unfavourable comparison with benefits in other European countries.
- The failure to provide paternity leave.
- The discrepancy between the length of minimum maternity leave and maternity pay.

Maternity pay coverage has improved but the higher SMP is still denied to the self-employed, and to women who earn less than £57 per week. Many of these women are in part-time work and low paid employment and often have greater needs than those women who are higher earners. The division between maternity pay and maternity allowance introduces a two-tier system of payment, even though the needs of pregnant women are similar.

The level of maternity pay compares unfavourably with other countries in the European Union. Maternity Alliance, an organization which campaigns for improvements in the rights and services for mothers, fathers and babies, issued a comparison between the benefits paid in the European Union countries and this is shown as figure 8.1. Maternity Alliance's eventual aim is for all working women to receive full pay during maternity leave.

Some European countries, notably Sweden, have introduced paternity leave entitlement to enable fathers to take some time off after the birth of their baby. Morris and Nott [1] suggest that the granting of parental leave, to be taken by either mother or father as they choose in order to meet their unique needs, may go some considerable way towards the elimination of stereotypical attitudes towards caring.

There is an argument that confining rights to time off from work to

| Comparison of Maternity Benefits in Europe (maternity pay expressed as a multiple of weekly earnings) | | |
|---|---|---|
| Country | Statutory Pay | Equivalent No. of Weeks on Full Pay |
| Denmark | 28 weeks on 90% of salary | 22 weeks |
| Italy | 20 weeks on 80% of salary | 17 weeks |
| Luxembourg | 16 weeks on 100% of salary | 16 weeks |
| Greece | 16 weeks on 100% of salary | 16 weeks |
| Netherlands | 16 weeks on 100% of salary | 16 weeks |
| Germany | 14 weeks on 100% of salary | 14 weeks |
| France | 16 weeks on 84% of salary | 13.5 weeks |
| Spain | 16 weeks on 75% of salary | 12 weeks |
| Belgium | 4 weeks on 82% and 10 weeks on 75% of salary | 11 weeks |
| Ireland | 14 weeks on 70% of salary | 10 weeks |
| United Kingdom | 6 weeks on 90% of salary and 12 weeks at £52.50 | 8 weeks |

**Fig. 8.1** A comparison of maternity benefit levels in the European Union.

women only can act as a form of discrimination against women in the development of their careers, and that this may be minimized if the time taken off for early child rearing is shared between mother and father to a greater extent than is possible at the moment.

There is a curious anomaly in the changes introduced in 1994. Although SMP is payable for 18 weeks, the shorter maternity leave entitlement is only 14 weeks and cannot be extended. For those women who receive only minimum entitlement to leave, this means that they cannot receive four weeks of their SMP. This tends to disadvantage the less well off as they are more likely to be working for employers who do not provide an occupational maternity benefit scheme. These latter schemes usually exceed the minimum state benefits, including offering extended leave arrangements. Women in these schemes can then receive the maximum SMP payments.

### Occupational maternity benefits

Many employers, particularly the larger companies and public sector organizations, offer occupational maternity benefits. There is no statutory obligation to do so but the schemes improve upon the minimum state provided benefit. These organizations claim back reimbursement to the level of SMP and then 'top up' their employee's salary to the level agreed in their scheme.

# NON-MATERNITY BENEFITS

## Income Support and Family Credit

These are two statutory benefits which are generally available. They are not pregnancy related but do provide important benefits to women who are on low wages. Both are means tested benefits and provide a 'safety net' payment to people on low income. Family Credit is paid to a family when one parent is working at least 24 hours per week. Income Support is paid to someone who is working less than 24 hours and tops up other benefits that may be received.

Entitlement to Income Support is graduated. The young person under 16 may not receive any payment. Usually between 16 and 18 years there is no entitlement although a young woman who is pregnant may apply for the benefit 11 weeks before her baby is due and for the six weeks afterwards. There are also two payment levels, a lower level paid to the under-25s and a higher level paid to the over-25s.

Maternity Alliance made representation to the House of Commons Select Committee chaired by Nicholas Winterton that the pregnant woman should receive the higher amount regardless of her age. In the 1992 report on *Maternity Services* the committee observed:

'It seems to us that a pregnant 24-year old is no different from a pregnant 26-year old and should not get significantly different amounts of benefit, let alone 16 and 17-year olds.'

The Government's point of view was also put to the Committee:

'... there were two rates of benefits, householders and non-householders. That was obviously not something that we wanted to continue. It was decided that in order to help the people who had the greatest expenses, who were the over-25s, these differential rates would apply. It was also true that the Government of the day had incentives very much in mind and that for younger people one did not want to construct a benefit system which would encourage people not to seek work ... The under-25s had fewer family responsibilities and were much more likely to be living with family and friends and did not have the expense of fully independent living.' [2]

The House of Commons Committee recommended that pregnant 18

to 24-year olds who qualify for Income Support should have it paid at the full adult rate. The Government in its response rejected this recommendation.

## The Social Fund

This fund was set up to provide a package of loans and one-off payments for those who can show they need help with specific expenditures. Related to maternity care, it replaces the universal maternity benefit payment that was intended to meet some of the initial costs of having a baby, although its value had, by the time of its abolition, been severely eroded. The new payment is means tested and available to those receiving Income Support or Family Credit. Payment is to a maximum of £100 and is reduced if the woman has savings over £500. Application for this assistance can be made after the twenty ninth week of pregnancy and can be claimed if the baby is born alive or stillborn after this time. The woman must apply to the local Department of Social Security and submit Form MAT B1, signed by the doctor or midwife. After the birth, she must then submit a second form, MAT B2, within three months of the delivery.

The Select Committee also considered the level of this fund. It drew attention to the abolition of special supplementary benefits which were available to a maximum of £187 and which were withdrawn with the introduction of the Social Fund. Effectively, it concluded, there had been a significant reduction in the level of benefit, and it recommended research into the cost of having a baby so that the Social Fund payments might be set at a more realistic level.

## MATERNITY BENEFITS – THE IMPLICATIONS FOR MIDWIFERY PRACTICE

The introduction to this chapter suggested that midwives can play a key role in assisting women to understand and obtain the benefits that they are statutorily entitled to. In one small administrative respect their help is vital – signing the Form MAT B1 – as many of the benefits and allowances are dependent upon the production of this.

Social security payments, maternity leave and allowances can nevertheless be complicated and some women will need specialist advice to obtain maximum assistance.

(1) Some local councils employ Welfare Rights Officers whose expertise is in helping people through the Social Security 'maze'.

(2) Where Welfare Rights Officers are not available the Citizens Advice Bureaux also have considerable experience in this field.

(3) Social workers and health visitors are obvious professionals who may also be able to help a woman if her claim is complicated.

If it is clear that a woman is having financial difficulties and does not appear to be getting the help she should, referral to any of these agencies should be considered.

# THE STATUTORY RIGHT TO MATERNITY CARE

## The right to a midwife's care

'A midwife may not, in law, refuse to give midwifery care to a woman if it is needed.'

This is a common misinterpretation of the legal obligation of midwives towards pregnant woman. There is nothing in the statutory governance of midwives that imposes this level of responsibility but, to illustrate where obligations begin and end, look at the following situations:

(1) Carol is in independent practice. She is currently caring for twenty women and would like, if possible, to plan a summer holiday. Gillian, who is ten weeks pregnant, comes to her clinic and asks to book with Carol. Carol explains that she is not taking any more bookings for the moment and gives Gillian the name and address of another independent midwife, the name and address of the supervisor of midwives and also advises her to go to her general practitioner.

(2) Louise is a community midwife working for an NHS maternity service. She works with two other midwives in a small team that holds a caseload which is currently full. Lisa comes to one of her clinics and asks to book with the team. Louise explains that she cannot take any more bookings at the moment and refers her to another local group of midwives.

Both situations are very similar and in both cases the midwives have apparently 'refused' care, even though for very good reasons. There is an obvious difference in that Carol is self-employed and Louise is employed by the NHS. In fact neither of them has a statutory obligation to provide care but Louise, as an employee of the NHS, probably has the greater obligation.

The main statutory obligation is one that is placed upon the NHS. Under the Health Service Act 1977, the Secretary of State has a duty

'to provide throughout England and Wales, to such an extent as he considers necessary to meet all reasonable requirements ... such other facilities for the care of expectant and nursing mothers and young children as he considers are appropriate as part of the health service.'

Under that requirement, and as an 'agent' of the NHS, Louise has an absolute obligation to ensure that Lisa will have maternity care, even if she cannot do it herself. If she fails to find another midwife she should continue to give care to Lisa. Although Carol would have a professional obligation to give Gillian advice on how to get maternity care, she does not have an absolute obligation to ensure that Gillian finds suitable support.

## The right to a general practitioner's care

All people have the right to general practitioner services but the obligation to provide these to the population rests not with individual general practitioners but with the Family Health Services Authorities (FHSAs). Most people of course are accepted onto the list of the general practitioner of their choosing, but, if they cannot find one, the FHSA must ensure that they are registered with a family doctor. Occasionally this registration is temporary and passes from one general practitioner to the next in rotation.

Maternity care is provided under a fee-for-services arrangement additional to the *per capita* payment which is related to the number of people on a general practitioner's list. General practitioners may decide that they do not want to provide all or part of maternity care, or the woman may wish to chose a different general practitioner for her maternity care.

If this is the case, the woman who has a right to maternity care should expect the FHSA to find another doctor to look after her. Because this second doctor would not be her general practitioner, he must be on the Obstetric List. He would then receive the fee for maternity care. Although a doctor may choose not to provide routine care and cannot be forced to do so, he cannot refuse to respond to an emergency call, including a request to attend a woman in labour if something is going wrong.

As well as having a right to general practitioner services, even if not always from her own general practitioner, the woman also has the right not to book a general practitioner to give her care.

Some women expressly ask not to see a doctor when pregnant and may just book a midwife. In fact there is no legal obligation on a woman to have any professional help when pregnant or in labour. All the statutory obligations rest with the health service, the moral and ethical obligations with the professionals and a statutory prohibition on everyone who is not a midwife or doctor against attending a woman in childbirth.

In practice, one of the situations that can create difficulty for the midwife and the woman she is looking after is the decision of the general practitioner not to offer maternity care. This is commonly related to the woman's request to have a homebirth. The FHSA cannot mandate the general practitioner to provide care but it is responsible for finding an alternative if the doctor refuses such care and the woman wants medical cover. The midwife should always refer these difficulties to her supervisor of midwives.

## SUMMARY

Statutory financial benefits for pregnant women are Statutory Maternity Pay and Maternity Allowance. They may also have grants up to £100 from the Social Fund.

There are varying lengths of statutory maternity leave. All working women have the right to a minimum of 14 weeks leave. Non-statutory occupational schemes common in the public sector and larger firms often improve upon the state provided minimum.

Income Support and Family Credit are generally available to those who are not in full-time work or who are on very low incomes.

Women also have the statutory right to receive maternity care and the absolute obligation to provide it rests with the NHS. Professional obligation to provide care relies upon professional responsibility and accountability rather than statutory obligation.

## FURTHER ACTION

- Invite an officer of the Department of Social Security to the unit to explain the changes to the Maternity Benefits which have taken place as a result of the European Directive.

- Write to the Maternity Alliance, 15 Britannia Street, London WC1X 9JP to obtain their leaflet on maternity benefits.

- Discuss with colleagues the continuing exclusion of some women from the benefit system and what midwives can do about it.

- See whether there is a current local procedure to cover the times when a woman appears not to have medical cover for her maternity care.

## REFERENCES

1. Morris, A.E. and Nott, S.M. *Working Women and the Law: equality and discrimination in theory and practice.* London, Routledge/Sweet and Maxwell, 1991.

2. Parliamentary Report of the House of Commons Health Committee. *Maternity Services.* Second Report, Session 1991–92, Vol. 1. London, HMSO, 1992.

# Chapter 9
# A Miscellany of Statutes

This chapter outlines the main provisions of some of the Acts of Parliament that have a bearing on midwifery practice.

The past thirty years have seen significant changes in moral and ethical attitudes which have affected human reproduction. Alongside this, there have been outstanding advances in medical science which have pushed forward the boundaries of clinical practice, particularly in the fields of genetics and assisted reproduction. The legal framework for dealing with some of the contentious issues that have been created by these advances is still developing. Some legislation, like the Abortion Act 1967, is well established even if still controversial; other legislation is fairly new and the extent of its influence has yet to be assessed. This includes the Surrogacy Arrangements Act 1985 and the Human Fertilisation and Embryology Act 1990.

Finally the chapter briefly introduces the main principles of the Children Act 1989 and covers Adoption.

## REPRODUCTIVE ETHICS

### The Abortion Act 1967

This Act was brought to Parliament as a Private Members' Bill. The Act allows for legal abortion by confirming that a registered medical practitioner will not be found guilty of an offence if he carries out an abortion under the requirements of the Act.

These are that two registered medical practitioners must be of the opinion, formed in good faith (although in an emergency only one doctor's opinion will be enough):

- that the pregnancy has not exceeded its twenty-fourth week and that the continuance of the pregnancy would involve risk, greater than if the pregnancy were terminated, of injury to the physical or mental health of the pregnant woman or any existing children of her family; or

- that the termination is necessary to prevent grave permanent injury to the physical or mental health of the pregnant woman; or

- that the continuance of the pregnancy would involve risk to the life of the pregnant woman, greater than if the pregnancy were terminated; or

- that there is a substantial risk that if the child were born it would suffer from such physical or mental abnormalities as to be seriously handicapped.

The abortion must be carried out in a licensed establishment if it is not done in an NHS hospital and the doctors must comply with the regulations regarding proper notification of the abortion.

Anyone who does not wish to be involved in legal termination of pregnancy may declare their conscientious objection. The responsibility for proving this rests with the individual; in Scotland, a statement of objection made in a Court will be accepted as such proof.

### Implications in practice

Some maternity services have extended their sphere of responsibility to cover all aspects of pregnancy related care including the legal termination of pregnancy. In other services, maternity and gynaecology are managed together and midwives are occasionally required to work in the gynaecology wards. In the community they may already be involved in giving antenatal care to a woman when it is decided she should have a termination of pregnancy.

Midwives are trained in giving support to women when they have had a stillbirth or neonatal death and this puts them in a unique position to offer support to women who also lose their pregnancy through termination. It is only involvement in the actual abortion for which they can claim conscientious objection, and not the care before and after the procedure.

If the midwife has an objection she should notify this at the earliest possible moment. This is probably advisable on taking up a new appointment so that the management can make arrangements for her objections to be honoured. This need to report an objection as early as possible is required by the UKCC in its guidance *Professional Conduct*. The nurse or midwife should

'report to an appropriate person or authority, at the earliest possible time, any conscientious objection which may be relevant to [her] professional practice.' [1]

## Surrogacy Arrangements Act 1985

It is estimated that between 10 and 15% of couples are infertile. Although advances in medical science have offered hope of having children to some of these, there are couples who still cannot be helped. With the development of extra-corporeal fertilization, an understandable next step for these couples was to arrange for another woman to carry a child for them.

In the mid-1980s a few cases were widely reported.

> In the case of Baby Cotton an American couple paid an English woman to be inseminated with the man's semen. The couple came to England to take the baby back to the United States but, following considerable media attention, the local authority made the child a ward of court and asked for a ruling on the future of the child.

The judge decided, based on his view of the best interests of the child, that the American couple could take it back to the United States. The judge however expressed his concerns about the commercial aspects of the case as money had been given to the surrogate mother and an agency had been involved in the arrangement.

Parliament acted after this case and introduced the Surrogacy Arrangements Act 1985. This Act makes it illegal for surrogacy to be arranged commercially in the UK. There should be no agency involvement and no fee can be paid. It also states that any surrogacy arrangement is unenforceable so that the woman who has the child cannot be forced to give it up, neither can the receiving couple be forced to take it.

Courts which may be called upon to adjudicate in a dispute arising from a surrogacy arrangement would be expected to make the decision based, as in the Baby Cotton case, in the best interests of the child. A midwife or doctor assisting a surrogacy arrangement in any way will not be guilty of a criminal offence unless they contravene the terms of the Act.

There are still many issues relating to surrogacy that the Act has not addressed. These include what to do if either party changes her mind about the arrangement and whether payment of expenses is excluded from the ban on money changing hands. Future cases may need to be referred to the courts for clarification.

A midwife may find herself involved in surrogacy if she has to look after the woman who is carrying the child. Her position is quite clear. She has a professional duty to give care and will not be committing a criminal act.

She should discuss the postnatal support for the child as it may be transferred immediately to the commissioning couple. If possible, discussions should take place with them about the postnatal care of the child, so that the midwives in the place where the child is to go can be informed and can arrange for postnatal care. This will need to be done efficiently so that the child can have the early metabolic screening tests.

Both the biological mother and the commissioning couple should be assured of the confidential nature of the referral from one midwife to another, but if they refuse to give details of their future address the midwife should discuss this with her supervisor and write a statement about the circumstances of the case.

# The Human Fertilisation and Embryology Act 1990

As medical technologies to assist conception developed, they began to raise ethical and moral issues so that in the early 1980s a committee was set up to examine all aspects of assisted reproduction and to report. The report of the Committee of Enquiry into Human Fertilisation and Embryology (The Warnock Report) was published in 1984. It was lengthy and detailed but its main recommendation was that legislation should be passed setting up a statutory licensing authority which would regulate matters related to infertility services and research.

### The HFEA

The Human Fertilisation and Embryology Act 1990 set up the Human Fertilisation and Embryology Authority (the HFEA) with the following general functions.

(1) To keep under review information about embryos and any subsequent development of embryos and about the provision of treatment services and activities governed by the Act and to advise the Secretary of State.

(2) To publicize its services.

(3) To provide advice and information.

(4) To issue a Code of Practice giving guidance about the proper conduct of activities carried on in pursuance of a licence under the Act and including guidance on the welfare of children born as a result of treatment services and any other children who may be affected by such births.

(5) To issue licences to those whose activities require a licence under the Act, notably for treatment services, storage and research purposes.

The Act defines treatment services as 'medical, surgical or obstetric services provided to the public or a section of the public for the purpose of assisting women to carry children'. The woman will not be seen as carrying a child until the embryo has become implanted. Specific treatments that must be licensed include donor insemination, in vitro fertilization, gamete intra-fallopian transfer, zygote intra-fallopian transfer and ovum donation.

## Artificial insemination

The Act also outlines the legal relationship of the mother and father when artificial insemination by donor has occurred.

- The woman who carries the child is legally the mother whether or not her own or a donor ovum is used.

- If her partner consents to artificial insemination by donor, then he is accepted as the father of the child.

- A donor is never legally recognized as the parent.

## Ovum donation

In its capacity as 'watchdog' over a rapidly changing technology, the HFEA constantly monitors developments and from time to time conducts a public consultation with a view to suggesting amendments to the law. For example, there had been growing concern about the lack of potential donors of ova so that the waiting lists of couples awaiting treatment that requires ovum donation had grown. It had been suggested that ova could be harvested from fetal ovaries when abortion has occurred. This raised major ethical questions, particularly about the parentage of the subsequent child.

In 1993 the HFEA issued a public consultation document to assess reaction to the use of fetal material in assisted reproduction. As well as being available in public libraries, it was circulated to all the relevant professional organizations including the Royal College of Midwives. (It is through such circulations that midwives are able to make comment and perhaps influence legislation.)

In July 1994, the HFEA published its recommendations following this consultation period. Principally for the sake of the children born by such means, it banned the use of ova from a fetus or from a dead woman in the treatment of infertility. It agreed that this material could be used for research purposes provided the woman having a termination consented to its use or the woman who died had previously consented. The research project for which this material is intended must also be approved by the HFEA.

# THE CHILDREN ACT 1989

This Act brings together the comprehensive law relating to children. It defines the rights of children, identifies the responsibilities of parents, makes provision for various 'care' and supervision orders and sets out procedures to be adopted for the protection of children.

## Child centred

Central to the Act is the paramount consideration of the welfare of the child in all court decisions and the ideal that these decisions should be made with minimum delay. Where possible, the child's own wishes and feelings about the future should be heard. The court should also take account of:

- physical, emotional and educational needs;
- age, sex, and background;
- any harm the child has suffered or is at risk of suffering; and
- how capable the parents or any other relevant person is of meeting the child's needs.

If the court is considering making an order in respect of the child, it should first consider whether it is better not to make an order at all.

## Parental responsibility

Parental responsibility is defined.

- When the parents are married to each other at the time of the child's birth they have joint responsibility.

- The mother has sole responsibility when she is not married.

- If not married to the mother the father does not have parental responsibility but he may apply to the court for an order granting him parental responsibility.

- Alternatively, the father and mother may by agreement (a parental responsibility agreement) provide for the father to have parental responsibility for the child.

## Court orders

In family proceedings a contact order or a residence order may be granted. The **contact order** requires the person with whom the child lives to allow the child to have contact with another named person. A

**residence order** settles the arrangements over where the child is to reside.

The court can also make **care** and **supervision orders** placing the child in the care of a designated local authority. These orders may be granted if the court is satisfied that the child is suffering or is likely to suffer significant harm, or that inadequate care is being given, or if the child is beyond parental control.

Child assessment orders and emergency protection orders are designed to protect the child. The **child assessment order** requires that the person with whom the child resides makes the child available for assessment, but in normal circumstances the child will remain at home. In making such an order, the court must be satisfied that the child does not need the protection of an emergency protection order. If the child is of sufficient age and understanding he is able to refuse to submit to an assessment order.

The **emergency protection order** may be made if the child is likely to suffer significant harm if not removed to accommodation provided by the applicant (commonly the local authority). When granting an emergency order the court can determine what contact the child will have with his parents, what medical or other examinations he should have and when it would appear safe to return him.

The midwife can be in a unique position to assess the well-being of children as she usually has unrestrained access to women's homes. Her informal surveillance of the well-being of all the children in a household may be the first opportunity to identify suspected child abuse or neglect. If she does have suspicions, she should report them to her supervisor, her manager and to the family's general practitioner. The family should be referred to the Social Services Department who should rapidly investigate the circumstances and take necessary action.

Fortunately the protective systems for children usually work well and it is the exception that results in an adverse outcome. However when children are harmed even though the health and social services agencies are involved, poor communication between professionals is often found to be a factor. It is good midwifery practice to follow up any verbal report in writing and, if no action is taken, to make further urgent contact about the child's situation.

Health authorities and local authority social services departments have been required to put processes in place to ensure that child protection arrangements are unequivocal. Staff, including midwives, should have training in these procedures and each health authority should designate an officer responsible for child protection matters including staff training and liaison with other agencies concerned in the protection of children.

# ADOPTION

The law on adoption is set out in the Adoption Act 1976 and the Adoption (Scotland) Act 1978, with amendments in the Children Act 1989 which bring the provisions of the two original Acts into line with the 1989 Act.

Adoption severs the legal relationship between a child and its natural parent(s) and creates a new legal relationship between the child and its adoptive parents. The overriding principle in any adoption process is that the child's welfare must always remain paramount and, to ensure that the child is protected, the legislation is very detailed in how and when an adoption can take place and who may adopt.

## Who may adopt and be adopted?

When two people adopt a child they must be married and, if neither is the parent of the child, they must both be over 21. If one of the couple is the natural parent, then only one needs to be 21. A single person, again over 21, may adopt.

The child to be adopted must be under 18 and not married or previously adopted.

## The process of adoption

All local authorities must provide an adoption service which offers advice, provides social work support when necessary and may also act as an adoption agency. There are also private and charitable adoption agencies, all of which must be registered with the local authority. These agencies arrange the adoption, acting as intermediaries between the parties, ensuring that the legal requirements are met and, most importantly, ensuring that the child's interests are protected.

When an adoption is to take place, the first thing that must happen is that the child's natural parent frees the child for adoption. She may not do this until the child is six weeks old and a child will not be placed with the adoptive parents until this has happened. When the child is in the care of the local authority and there is no prospect of returning to his natural parent, the local authority may make an application to waive this requirement.

When a child is placed with adoptive parents, it must be with them for at least 13 weeks prior to the granting of an adoption order and a child must be at least 19 weeks old before such an order will be granted.

During this time, extensive enquiries are made about the suitability of the parents, and their growing relationship with the child is assessed by social workers of the adoption agency. A 'guardian ad litem' is also appointed for the child. This is an officer of the court, whose responsibility it is to draw together everything that is known about the investigations as well as to ensure that the legal processes are properly completed. One important step is to ensure that the putative father is not going to apply for parental responsibility or a residence order.

All this is done on the child's behalf and the guardian finally compiles a report for the court with a recommendation about what the court should decide. If the recommendation is that adoption is in the interests of the child the court will issue an Adoption Order, and the adoption will have taken place.

## Access to birth registration information

Since 1975 it has been possible for an adopted person to apply to the Registrar General for information that will enable him to obtain his original birth certificate. This will show the name and address of his natural mother as it was at the time of registration. A counselling service is available for people who want this information and, for people who were adopted before 12 November 1975, they must have counselling first.

The Children Act 1989 has introduced a further measure to facilitate contact between adopted people and their natural parents. The Registrar General now keeps an Adoption Contact Register. It is in two parts. On Part 1, adopted people who wish to make contact with natural relatives may place their name and address. Relatives who wish to make contact with an adopted person place their name and address on Part 2. An administration fee is paid for this service.

## SUMMARY

Legislation relating to human reproduction is contained in the Abortion Act 1967, the Human Fertilisation and Embryology Act 1990 and the Surrogacy Arrangements Act 1985. These issues often raise ethical and moral questions which are the subject of public consultation from time to time. Midwives are in a unique position to contribute to such consultation.

Child welfare and protection legislation is provided by the Children Act 1989. Midwives should be aware of the local arrangements that have been devised to ensure that children have immediate protection if it is required.

Adoption is covered in the Adoption Acts and Children Act 1989. In any adoption proceedings, the interests of the child are paramount and the legal requirements for the adoption process support this principle.

## FURTHER ACTION

- Write to your professional association asking for details of its response to the 1993 public consultation on the use of donated fetal gametes.

- Find out who is the responsible officer for child protection matters where you work.

- If you have not seen them, ask for a copy of the local guidelines to staff on child protection and find out why you have not seen them.

## REFERENCE

1. United Kingdom Central Council for Nursing, Midwifery and Health Visiting. *Code of Professional Conduct for the Nurse, Midwife and Health Visitor*, London, UKCC, 1992.

# Chapter 10
# Employment Matters

Most midwives are employees with almost all of them working for the NHS. Because employment law is not specific to midwifery this chapter only summarizes the main provisions of current employment law. These are found in the Employment Protection (Consolidation) Act 1978, amended in subsequent employment legislation in the 1980s.

Midwifery is a female dominated profession and women, often working women, are their clients. The chapter, therefore, discusses the law on sex discrimination and the extent to which statutory protection is successful in achieving equality of opportunity.

A few midwives are self-employed. There are about a hundred midwives in independent practice at present, but this number may increase as maternity services provision becomes more flexible. There are particular legal obligations that relate to self-employment and others that apply if the midwife employs someone in her practice.

## BEING EMPLOYED

### The contract of employment

A contract exists between an employer and employee whether or not it is in writing and the principles of the contract rely upon common law rather than statute. The employer has the right to expect the employee to do his job and in return the employee has the right to expect fair treatment by the employer, including a reasonable remuneration for his work. A contract exists from the day when an employee begins work and any terms and conditions agreed upon will form part of that contract. If either party breaks the terms of the contract they can sue for breach of contract. This can be a very costly way of seeking redress so it is rarely used now.

The statutory provisions of the 1978 Act are additional to these common law principles. Employees who work eight hours or more each week are entitled to receive a written statement of the main terms and conditions of their employment. This should include:

- the names of employer and employee,
- the date when employment began,
- the remuneration,
- the hours of work,
- holiday and sick leave entitlement,
- pension arrangements,
- notice of termination arrangements,
- job title,
- the length of any fixed term contract job,
- the place of work and
- any collective agreements which apply to the post.

Details of disciplinary and grievance procedures should also be included if the firm has over 20 employees.

The collective agreements that apply to the NHS are made by the Whitley Councils. There are general conditions which apply to all NHS workers and further specific agreements made by functional councils for groups of workers. The agreements relating to midwives are made by the Nursing and Midwifery Staffs Negotiating Council.

Until the passing of the National Health Service and Community Care Act 1990, these agreements applied in all NHS establishments. The Act enabled the newly formed NHS Trusts to develop their own terms and conditions of service, although they are not bound to do so. As a result there is now a varying pattern of terms and conditions within the NHS. Some Trusts still use the national agreements in their totality, some have developed their own terms including new pay scales, while others have used a mixture of the national agreements and their own terms to form unique employment contracts.

Added to this greater flexibility of contract terms, the national agreements are now often 'enabling' agreements rather than binding terms. That is, they outline possible entitlements, but then leave it to the local employer to decide whether to implement them. There is, for example, an enabling agreement for paternity and adoption leave. Some Trusts have incorporated these into their employees' contracts, others have not.

There has been considerable suspicion of this greater flexibility. It is possible that local Trusts will use it to hold wages down, particularly if there are no local recruitment problems, and there is some evidence that this has happened, especially in unskilled or low skilled work. It can, however, allow for flexibility upwards if particular skills are in short supply.

The changes envisaged in the report, *Changing Childbirth*, will require midwives to adopt more flexible working patterns and take on greater personal accountability. The report acknowledges that as this happens midwives' remuneration should reflect their greater responsibility levels and this will only be achieved if there is local pay flexibility.

## Other statutory employment rights

Many of the rights conferred by legislation only apply when an employee has completed a qualifying period. This is two years full-time employment (16 hours or over per week) or five years part-time employment (8 to 16 hours per week). Movement within the NHS counts as continuity of employment.

Other employment rights include:

- the right to an itemized payslip,
- the right to belong to a trade union,
- the right to reasonable time off with pay for trade union duties if the employee is a union official,
- the right to time off with pay for safety representatives to fulfil their duties,
- the right to time off (but not paid time) for certain public duties, including being a Justice of the Peace and membership of statutory tribunals or authorities, and
- the right to reasonable time off to look for work if made redundant.

Statutory rights when a job comes to an end include:

- the right of both the employer and employee to give or receive notice of termination of employment,
- the right, if dismissed, to receive written details of the reason on request,
- the right not to be unfairly dismissed, and
- if redundant, the right to redundancy payment.

## Wrongful dismissal

Under common law, the relationship between an employer and employee is that of two parties who have entered a contract. If either party repudiates the contract or fails to meet the terms of the contract, the other may claim breach of contract and claim damages. Effectively this used to be the only remedy open to employees who were summarily dismissed, but they were often in a weak position and it was rare for them to receive recompense. It was because of this unsatisfactory state of affairs that the first employment protection legislation was introduced in 1971.

The employment legislation is additional to the common law remedies, which can be used but rarely are. Very occasionally when an employee has been dismissed, application is made for an injunction to stop or delay the dismissal. This is usually used to enforce a proper period of notice to allow the employee time to invoke the statutory processes. Also very occasionally an injunction can be sought to stop an employer from unilaterally changing a substantive term of the contract.

## Unfair dismissal

Employees' rights on dismissal are, as with the other rights in this chapter, covered by the 1978 Act and its amendment in 1980. An employee who has been continuously employed either full- or part-time under the meaning of the Act, has the right not to be unfairly dismissed. If she believes this has happened she may apply to an industrial tribunal to seek redress.

In looking at the case, the tribunal will consider whether the reason for the dismissal was fair and whether it should have resulted in dismissal or a lesser form of sanction.

For the dismissal to be fair it should relate to:

- the employee's capacity or qualifications to do the job,
- to conduct,
- to redundancy, or
- to a legal restriction which prevents employment.

For an example of the last point, if a midwife is removed from the UKCC Register it would be fair to dismiss her as she can no longer practise legally.

Certain other circumstances will automatically be construed as unfair dismissal. These include dismissal because of membership of a trade union, or because of undertaking trade union duties, and dismissal on grounds of pregnancy. This latter provision has been considerably strengthened by the changes discussed in Chapter 8.

If the Industrial Tribunal finds that the employee has been unfairly dismissed it may make one of three orders.

- **Re-instatement**. The employee goes back to his original job as though he had not been dismissed.
- **Re-engagement**. The employee is offered a new job by his employer.
- **Compensation**. The employee does not return to work but instead receives compensation calculated on a similar basis to redundancy and with an additional sum to compensate for the loss of the job.

To minimize the possibility of an unfair dismissal claim, personnel departments take great care over the procedures that they adopt when disciplining staff. In the NHS these procedures usually take the form of an initial hearing with the employee having the right to appeal to her employing authority or Trust. A midwife finding herself faced with any form of disciplinary action should make immediate contact with her trade union for support. The processes can be very complex and daunting, and on her own she may fail to obtain the redress to which she is statutorily due.

# Discrimination on grounds of sex

### Movements towards equality

In 1970 the Equal Pay Act was passed. This required that men and women who are employed in like work should receive the same pay and conditions of service.

However this Act did not redress the balance of remuneration as had been hoped. Under the Act, a woman had to compare her position with men undertaking substantially the same job. This ignored one of the main difficulties faced by women: they were employed in low paid women's work for which there were no comparators. Secretaries, for example, were almost exclusively women and so were unable to question the wage differentials between them and male colleagues of similar status doing different work.

In 1974, a challenge to this position was launched by referring to a section of the Treaty of Rome, Article 119. This states that:

> 'Each member state shall . . . maintain the application of the principle that men and women should receive equal pay for equal work.'

A case in 1988, *Pickstone* v. *Freemans PLC* confirmed the right of women to use this directive in claims for equal pay and this course of action should be open to them even if some men were doing the same job.

The Sex Discrimination Act 1975 makes it generally unlawful for an employer to discriminate on grounds of sex or marriage. There are some limited exceptions to this but when the Act was passed it was not felt that midwifery should be one of these. Although it took some pilot schemes, and there were original restrictions, it was the passage of this Act that opened the profession to men.

### The EOC and discrimination in the NHS

The 1975 Act set up the Equal Opportunities Commission (EOC) with responsibility for monitoring sex discrimination and giving advice and active support to people (usually but not exclusively women) in discrimination claims. Their studies and evidence from many other sources confirm that equality of work opportunity for women is still some way off.

In 1990 the EOC undertook a study into equal opportunities policies in the NHS. It identified the NHS as the largest employer of women in Western Europe. The results of the study were published in 1991 as the report *Equality Management. Women's employment in the NHS* [1]. The study showed that discrimination still existed at every level of the organization, in all of the occupations in the service and in most of the personnel policies that they scrutinized. It also found that access to training was limited for women, largely because such opportunities were not available to part-time workers.

This discrimination is equally apparent in the traditional woman's job of nursing. A study of nursing career patterns carried out for the Department of Health and Social Services in 1986 [2] examined the length of time it took from initial qualification to reach nursing officer grade. The most striking finding of this study was that it took the men in the study an average of 8.4 years to achieve promotion whereas it took the women who had no career break 14.5 years. Discrimination existed even when women did not take time away from their career, a common reason given to explain poor career progression.

This is just one of many studies that indicate the existence of discrimination in relation to work opportunities despite the protection of UK and European legislation.

A major problem stems from the need to look at all claims on an individual basis and going to law on matters of principle which can be applied to other cases can be expensive. Like the case of Mrs Pickstone, such cases invariably need the backing of an organization like the EOC. Its funding is limited and it has to be careful therefore in its selection of cases to support.

This is probably one of the areas of law where change is best achieved by working at organizational level, ensuring that all policies are effective in eliminating discrimination, rather than expressly turning to the legal system. However, individuals who believe they have been discriminated against may seek redress at an industrial tribunal. It is usual in these circumstances to have the support of a trade union or professional organization.

## Discrimination on grounds of race

The Race Relations Act 1976 makes it generally unlawful for employers to discriminate on racial grounds. This includes race, colour, nationality, citizenship, and ethnic or national origins. The responsibility for monitoring the effectiveness of the legislation lies with the Commission for Racial Equality (CRE), which was set up under the 1976 legislation.

As well as monitoring discrimination and occasionally supporting legal cases of significance, the CRE has published a Code of Employment Practice. It is currently producing codes for specific areas of activity and in 1994 issued a new code of good practice for the NHS Maternity Services. This and the main code are available from the CRE.

## Indirect discrimination.

Indirect discrimination occurs when a requirement or condition for a job apparently applies equally to different groups (men and women or different racial groups) but the proportion able to comply of one of the groups is considerably smaller than the proportion of the other group or groups. Both the Sex Discrimination Act 1975 and the Race Relations Act 1996 make indirect discrimination illegal and the statutory requirements are very similar.

An example of indirect discrimination would be a redundancy agreement which made part-timers redundant before full-timers. It could be argued that part-time working applies equally to men and women. However, in a company with women largely occupying the part-time posts and men in full-time employment, women would be considerably disadvantaged.

Bourn and Whitmore [3] suggest that four questions should be asked to test for indirect discrimination.

(1) Has a requirement or condition been applied equally to both sexes or all racial groups?

(2) Is that requirement or condition one with which a considerably smaller number of women (or men) or persons of the racial group in question can comply than those of the opposite sex or persons not of that racial group?

(3) Is the requirement or condition justifiable irrespective of the sex, colour, race, nationality, ethnic or national origins of the person in question?

(4) Has the imposition of the requirement or condition operated to the detriment of the person who could not comply with it?

## THE SELF-EMPLOYED MIDWIFE

There are still very few midwives in independent practice. This may change as the services become more flexible and already midwives are negotiating honorary contracts to use NHS facilities for delivery. One practice is in the process of arranging to offer a full range of midwifery care under contract to NHS patients.

Being self-employed means that the midwife herself has to accept the statutory responsibilities which relate to employment rather than relying on an employer. These include:

- the legal basis for working arrangements with colleagues,
- payment of taxes and national insurance,
- provision of professional indemnity,
- the provision of safe premises, equipment and other products, and
- the legal obligations towards employees.

## Working with colleagues

For reasons of cover and professional support, most midwives in independent practice work together in small group practices. Some have expressly entered a legal partnership while others work in an informal association with each other.

The law on partnerships is substantially defined by the Partnership Act 1890. It defines a partnership as:

'The relationship which subsists between persons carrying on a business in common with a view to profit.'

Essentially, a partnership is a contract formed between a minimum of two people.

It may be expressly formed or may be implied. Thus if it can be inferred that two or more people are acting in a partnership then it will be treated as one. Thus a midwifery practice which operates corporately, all using the same name, letter-headings and premises and referring to 'my partners', may be regarded legally as a partnership even if one has not been formally entered into.

For midwives, the most important result of such an arrangement is that the partnership is regarded as a firm and all partners are agents of the firm. All are therefore both individually and collectively liable and can be sued in the name of the firm as well as in their own right. The following example shows how this works.

> Sheila, Natalie and Vicky work together in a practice they have called the Littletown Group Midwifery Practice. Natalie and Vicky have membership of an organization that offers them professional indemnity insurance. Sheila is not personally covered but one night fails to diagnose complications in labour and transfers her client late into hospital. Subsequently the woman's solicitors issue a writ against her because the baby is brain damaged. She has no assets. The solicitors then advise the woman to take out a writ against the practice collectively and against Natalie and Vicky as individuals. He advises his client that, although they had not entered a formal partnership agreement, the three midwives had implied that they

were working together. They had pooled their remuneration and taken a share of profit out of the practice as their income.

The three midwives could have arranged their working arrangements differently to avoid this by booking women individually and making cover arrangements on a 'sub-contracted' basis. They should also have made it clear that they were working from the same premises but were independently offering their services.

Alternatively they could have made it an absolute requirement that each midwife in the partnership must hold insurance cover and so can separately indemnify the practice. In normal circumstances the acts of a partner bind the firm and the other partners unless the partner clearly has no authority to act. If Sheila had been expressly required to hold insurance under the terms of the partnership and did not, the other midwives might be able to argue that she was acting without authority and avoid liability.

The membership of partnerships can change. Any member can retire although they will continue to be responsible for any debts that may have been incurred while they were working for the practice. New partners may join but only with the consent of all the existing partners.

A partnership may be terminated under the following circumstances:

- at the end of a fixed term, if the partnership was only to exist for a fixed period;
- at the end of a simple undertaking, if the partnership was set up expressly to complete a single task;
- after notice of dissolution from any of the partners, so long as all the partners are in agreement; or
- by a court order, if the dissolution is not agreed by all the partners.

Detailed advice on whether to set up a partnership is outside the scope of this book, but all midwives who are thinking of going into private practice should talk to a solicitor. It is important that the relationship on the question of professional liability is clear. If they do not want a formal partnership to exist, midwives working together must make sure that they do not effectively introduce arrangements which could imply that a partnership has been founded.

# Matters of safety

## *The Health and Safety at Work Act 1974*

There is a history of legislation controlling safety at work which spans the nineteenth and twentieth centuries. The latest and most comprehensive is the Health and Safety at Work Act 1974. This Act places responsibilities upon both employers and employees to ensure that people in work are protected. It lays down general duties the most important of which, for midwives, can be summarized as follows.

(1) An employer must take all reasonable and practical steps to protect the health, safety and welfare of his employees.

(2) An employer must take all reasonable steps to protect non-employees from risk.

(3) Employees must take reasonable care in work to protect the health and safety of themselves and others and must co-operate with their employers so they fulfil their duties under the Act.

All large establishments, such as NHS units, appoint a Safety Officer, usually a member of the personnel department, who formulates a safety policy for the unit. Trades unions appoint Health and Safety Representatives who inspect the premises and working practices to check that all risks are minimized. It is usual for these groups to meet together from time to time to review health and safety matters, audit any work accidents and review the organization's policies.

Of course the midwife in independent practice will not set up such an elaborate system. She must however be aware that the provisions of the Act apply equally to her and should therefore examine all her working practices and those of any colleagues or employees to ensure that she is complying with the Act.

Failure to comply is a criminal offence. The Health and Safety Executive, which was set up under the Act, may prosecute anyone who does not comply. In the first instance they usually issue notices requiring compliance, but anyone found guilty under the Act can be fined or imprisoned or both.

## The Occupiers' Liability Acts 1957 and 1984

Midwives in independent practice usually provide premises from which they offer their services. This may be an integral part of their home or may be separate. In either case they are legally bound by the Occupiers' Liability Act 1957 to exercise a common duty of care for the reasonable safety of all visitors. By the 1957 Act this only applied to people who were lawfully on the premises but in 1984 liability was extended to cover trespassers as well.

This duty of care includes the safety of furniture and other things on the premises. It is possible to avoid liability for damage to property by putting up a clear disclaimer. An example of this is the notice in car parks that says the owner is not liable for damage or loss of the car or any personal effects. Since 1977 it has not been possible to exclude liability for personal injury. Any notice claiming such exemption would be considered null and void.

### Product liability

People can be damaged by things they buy or acquire when receiving professional services. If a midwife gives a drug to a woman which subsequently turns out to be sub-standard and damages her, or if someone buys a faulty electric drill and is injured as a result, they have the right to sue someone for negligence.

But who? The manufacturer? The shopkeeper? The midwife?

In 1985 a European Directive on product liability placed liability with the manufacturer in the first place, then with the supplier and finally with the person in direct contact with the consumer, the shopkeeper or the midwife. This was followed up in the UK by the Consumer Protection Act 1987. This is an excellent protection for the end supplier of goods so long as they can prove who the supplier or manufacturer is.

It is therefore good practice to keep a careful record of the suppliers of all batches of drugs and all equipment used so that it can be traced back in the case of a claim. For drugs and equipment used in the care of the woman, she will in normal circumstances have three years to issue a writ, but in the case of a baby, this could be as long as 21 years. Midwives may get guidance about how long to keep product records from their local health service supplies department or pharmacy.

## Professional indemnity insurance

The self-employed midwife is personally responsible for her professional actions and does not enjoy the employers' contractual indemnity that her employed colleague has. Although she is liable to her clients there is no legal obligation upon her to to take out insurance to cover for malpractice claims, but there is an ethical and moral imperative to do so. Indemnity insurance is commonly provided as part of the subscription to a professional organization or trade union.

This situation may change in the future. In 1993 the Royal College of Midwives, which provided cover to most of the self-employed midwives, experienced severe difficulties in obtaining cover for that sector and it is not certain whether any organization will in future provide insurance for the self-employed. Midwives may, like their medical colleagues in private practice, have to find personal cover for themselves. Because midwifery and obstetrics are viewed as high risk by the insurance market, the premiums are likely to be high.

The level of cover a midwife provides forms part of the contract with the woman she is looking after. It is also likely to be a stipulation of the honorary contracts between midwife and the NHS. If there is a likelihood of a change in the amount of cover that can be secured this should be made explicit before a contract is agreed. Any subsequent change may be seen as a breach of contract. In the case of agreements with NHS hospitals this will probably result in withdrawal of the use of the facilities. If a change of the terms is unavoidable and could not have been anticipated, the midwife should make this immediately known to the other party to the contract who can then decide whether to accept the change or cancel the agreement.

## The midwife as employer

Independent practices may employ staff. These may be for secretarial support, for health care assistant support or, occasionally, they may directly employ a midwife.

All employers are bound by the provisions of statutory employment law and common law as briefly detailed earlier in this chapter. The midwife employing other staff must treat staff fairly, must not dismiss staff unfairly and must not discriminate on grounds of race or sex.

As an employer, she will also be legally responsible for the collection of income tax as PAYE, the collection of the employees' national insurance contributions and payment of the employers' contribution to the scheme. Even where a practice uses other self-employed people on a 'consultancy' basis, it may be held liable for the tax of these people if they fail to pay themselves. For this reason it may be more sensible to employ staff directly although the taxation advantages of doing this may need to be balanced against the possible vicarious liability for employed staff.

The midwife who employs someone will be vicariously liable for the negligent actions of her employee. If this is another midwife the financial implications of this may be considerable as any indemnity cover would need to extend to both midwives. The future configuration of professional indemnity is uncertain but any midwife who is considering employing another colleague should seek advice from her professional organization or from the practice's legal advisers.

## WORKING ABROAD

The midwife who works abroad must comply with the legal requirements of the country she has gone to. If the country has a system of registration she will also need to be registered. This applies equally to midwives who have trained abroad who wish to work in the UK. To register, contact should be made with the country's registering body to find out what the requirements are, although this information may be readily available from the international departments of the professional associations. The UKCC will also give advice about registration requirements abroad.

The 1983 Midwifery Directive introduced reciprocity across the European Union. Training requirements were standardized in the Directive and midwives have freedom of movement within the European Union although countries may still test for linguistic fluency.

## SUMMARY

Most midwives in the UK are employees of the NHS and have common law and statutory protections in work. Their contracts of employment usually contains some nationally agreed terms and conditions although these are less common with the introduction of new powers for NHS Trusts.

There are anti-discriminatory laws in force in the UK but there is evidence that they are not wholly successful in achieving parity between groups.

Some midwives are self-employed and may sometimes be employers of staff. They have the usual legal obligations of employers.

## FURTHER ACTION

- Obtain the series of free leaflets on employment protection that are available from the Department of Employment (from local Job Centres).

- Ask your local steward, if you have one, to show you the Whitley Council agreements for nurses, midwives and health visitors.

- Draw a diagram of the management structure in your unit/service and identify the proportion of men to women at each level. Then look at the ethnic mix of these managers. Is possible discrimination apparent?

## REFERENCES

1. Equal Opportunities Commission. *Equality Management: Women's Employment in the NHS*. London, EOC, 1991.
2. Davies, C. and Rosser, J. *Processes of Discrimination: a study of women working in the NHS*. London, DHSS, 1986.
3. Bourn, C. and Whitmore, J. *Race and Sex Discrimination*, 2nd edn, London, Sweet and Maxwell, 1993.

# Table of Cases

Note the following abbreviations are used:

A         Appeal (US system)
AC        Law Reports, Appeal Cases
All ER    All England Law Reports
BMJ       British Medical Journal
Ch        Law Reports Chancery
H & C     Hurlstone & Coltman
ICR       Industrial Court Reports
LGR       Knight's Local Government Reports
QB        Law Reports, Queen's Bench Division
WLR       Weekly Law Reports

# Table of Statutes

# Index